RHEUMATISM AND ARTHRITIS

Explains this common but distressing problem in simple terms and discusses practical natural ways which can be of immediate benefit to the sufferer.

RHEUMATISM AND ARTHRITIS

Natural remedies and nutritional advice
for the alleviation of these
painful conditions

Leonard Mervyn
B.Sc., Ph.D., C.Chem., F.R.S.C.

*Prepared and produced by the Editorial Committee
of Science of Life Books*

SCIENCE OF LIFE BOOKS
11 Munro Street, Port Melbourne, Victoria 3207

Fifteenth Edition, completely revised, enlarged
and reset 1986

© SCIENCE OF LIFE BOOKS 1986

*Registered at the G.P.O. Sydney
for transmission through the post
as a book*

Inquiries should be made to the publishers:
Lothian Publishing Company Pty. Ltd.
11 Munro Street, Port Melbourne, 3207

U.K. Distributors:
THORSONS PUBLISHING GROUP
Wellingborough, Northamptonshire
U.S.A Distributors:
THORSONS PUBLISHERS INC.
New York

National Library of Australia card number
and ISBN 0-909911-15-0

Printed and bound in Great Britain

Contents

Note to reader

Before following the self-help advice given in this book readers are earnestly urged to give careful consideration to the nature of their particular health problem, and to consult a competent physician if in any doubt. This book should not be regarded as a substitute for professional medical treatment, and whilst every care is taken to ensure the accuracy of the content, the author and the publishers cannot accept legal responsibility for any problem arising out of the experimentation with the methods described.

Foreword

Rheumatism and arthritis are not 'killer diseases' yet they probably account for more pain, more suffering and more lost working hours than any other disorder. They are not 'terminal disorders'; however, once established they are often difficult to overcome and in most sufferers the condition becomes steadily worse until the patient finally dies from old age or some other malady.

Over the years medicine has done practically nothing to prevent the onset of rheumatism and arthritis and has achieved very little by way of treatment. Treatment aimed at relieving pain has had a moderate degree of success but all too often with side effects which may be as disastrous for the sufferers as their original problem.

Rheumatism and arthritis have no respect for persons — old and young alike, men and women, people of different races and cultures are all potential victims. There does not appear to be one common cause and each individual sufferer appears to be uniquely affected. In some only one or two joints may be affected, in others whole groups of muscles, a complete limb, the spinal column or even the whole body can be attacked.

Over the centuries many 'cures' have been promoted and folk medicine contains numerous methods of treatment and recipes for remedies which promise relief to the sufferer. Undoubtedly in some cases the 'folk remedies' have helped individuals, but they have failed to provide a satisfactory solution to the problem for the vast majority of those afflicted.

What are the causes of rheumatism and arthritis? Some of the more common would probably include nutrition, infection, hormonal disturbances, allergies, trauma, intoxication, exposure to pollutants and chemicals, and our modern lifestyle which only too often shows little respect for the natural environment for which our bodies were created.

One of the most important causes is undoubtedly nutrition. Nutrition in this sense includes not only the food we eat (our diet) but what the body does with that food and how it utilizes it, which considerably broadens the effect nutrition can have on our bodies. The utilization of food and the elimination of waste products is equally as important as the food we eat. For example, it is little use supplementing a body with fat-soluble vitamins if that body has a liver or pancreatic problem which interferes with the absorption of fats. Similarly if the body cannot eliminate waste products efficiently a build up of toxins or 'autotoxaemia' will occur. In order for a corrective diet to be effective the body must be able to utilize that diet.

In our 'western type' diet there are a number of items which masquerade as food and which find their way into our food chain in a great variety of ways. These include white sugar, common salt, coffee, tea, artificial colouring, artificial flavouring and a host of chemical residues from agricultural and food processing practices. These substances interfere with the utilization of natural foods and in many cases are themselves harmful, causing allergies and other reactions which add to the original problem. The person who suffers with rheumatism or arthritis will do well to take notice of the old adage 'eat nothing that comes out of a packet or a can' and to eat only whole natural foods prepared in the home.

If we look at the situation in Australia, for example, where the vast majority of people in later life suffer from some form of rheumatism or arthritis, and we take note that one third of all meals are prepared or eaten away from the home, and that cane sugar and alcohol account for 25 per cent of all calories (energy) consumed by the population, it is little wonder that years spent following a lifestyle such as this produce so many arthritic and rheumatic sufferers in the over fifty age group in many Western European countries as well as in America.

Another cause is the excess consumption of red meats and refined carbohydrate foods (white flour, polished rice, white sugar etc.). These commonly-used foods all promote the formation of uric acid, an accumulation of which can be directly responsible for gout, rheumatism or arthritis. The control of uric acid formation and its elimination is one of the key factors in the treatment of rheumatism and arthritis.

Overweight is another problem. (Which causes a great deal of concern.) When people suffer from rheumatism or arthritis, their painful joints or muscles usually deter them from adequate exercise, and if they do not adapt their food intake to meet their reduced energy expenditure an increase in weight is inevitable. This increased weight places an additional burden on inflamed and aching joints and so aggravates the condition, particularly if the feet, knees or hips are involved. It is imperative that any effort to treat rheumatism and arthritis should not neglect the potential danger of overweight. (A companion Science of Life book *Lose Weight and Gain Health* can greatly assist those who wish to control their weight.)

Fatigue is another problem which plagues the sufferer. This is not only due to the lack of exercise resulting from the pain and discomfort but in many cases also to the faulty assimilation of essential nutrients. Here vitamin and mineral supplements can be of great benefit, so too can foods such as wheatgerm, brewer's yeast, yogurt and crude black molasses, all of which provide essential nutrients and also assist normal functions of the digestive organs.

One of the most popular forms of treatment is the use of liniments and analgesic rubs to relieve local pain in muscles and joints. This is usually effective to some extent on a short-term basis; however it can be made more effective if the neighbouring area is also treated. For example in treating a stiff neck not only should the neck receive attention but the liniment or cream should also be massaged into the muscles extending from the collar bone in the front to bottom of the shoulder blades at the back. This is because the muscles in this area are responsible for many neck movements. Similarly if the elbow is affected both the forearm and the upper arm should receive attention.

What of the future? Will a cure be found for

rheumatism and arthritis or will the situation continue as it has done for past centuries, with one remedy after another finding popularity only to be replaced in a few years by yet another? Whatever the answer it does little to help the sufferer right now, unlike this book which has been designed to do just that. It does not promise a miraculous cure or a programme guaranteed to banish rheumatism and arthritis forever; rather it seeks to explain the problem in simple terms and discuss some practical natural means which can be of immediate benefit to the sufferer.

WILLIAM KING D.O., D.C.
New South Wales

1
What is Rheumatism?

In the minds of the public the term rheumatism is generally used as a contraction of the term muscular rheumatism where one group of muscles is affected at a time such as muscles of the shoulder, neck, back, loins, arms or leg. A more loose popular definition of the word is simply aches, pains and possibly stiffness in the muscles, bones, ligaments and joints anywhere in the body. Put simply, rheumatism describes any aches and pains not arising from the heart, lungs, kidneys, intestines and other structures within the body.

Rheumatism, then, is an umbrella word that embraces aches and pains due to conditions ranging from a simple, sprained ankle to a severe rheumatoid arthritis which is a serious complaint. Even arthritis, which means inflammation of one or more joints, can be due to a wide variety of conditions ranging from German measles to rheumatoid arthritis. Arthritis should not be confused with *arthrosis* which means a condition of a joint which is due to degeneration or wear and tear rather than inflammatory changes, although these may add an extra complication in some cases.

How did the word rheumatism arise? Its origin lies in antiquity when it was thought that any unpleasant aches and pains were caused by one of the four cardinal 'humours' discharged from the blood into the muscles and joints. The word 'rheum' in ancient Latin and Greek meant a flow of watery discharge, a kind of ugly catarrh flowing into the tissues and carrying disease into them. Now we know that this actually happens in the condition of gout where uric acid may pass from the blood and crystallize out in the joints causing agonizing pain. When, later in this book, we look at the explanations of natural diets and treatments that can relieve and even cure the complaint, perhaps we shall see that our ancestors may have had the right ideas about rheumatism and its causes.

It is likely that all of us have had or will have rheumatism at some time in our lives. Despite being an unpleasant, annoying and tedious complaint, rheumatism is rarely serious and seldom affects general health.

The symptoms need not indicate a serious condition. It is often caused by a cold draught, or a chill, which constricts the blood vessels in the affected region. This means the toxic matter in that region is not eliminated, and inflammation is set up. This localized condition calls for simple, local treatment, and usually passes after copious sweating has been induced (see p. 101).

Aches, Pains and Strains
We shall first look at the simpler conditions which produce pain and see how they may arise and be treated.

Leg cramps induced by walking

These cramps occur in the calf muscles and come on only after walking a certain distance. After rest they disappear only to reappear after walking a similar distance. The condition is known as 'intermittent claudication' and is a result of narrowing of the leg arteries. It is one of the few diseases that can be treated successfully just by a daily intake of between 400 and 600 i.u. of vitamin E.

Leg cramps in the night

In cramp the muscles bunch up and can be felt as hard, firm lumps. Relief is usually obtained by massaging the legs, getting out of bed and standing, or by simply moving the limbs which will make the painful hard muscular contractions quickly disappear. These cramps are sometimes associated with varicose veins and in these cases relief is achieved by raising the bottom of the bed a foot or so. This has the effect of allowing the blood to flow away from the legs and so reducing the swollen veins which in turn alleviates the pain. Night cramps are extremely common and may occur in healthy people of any age, even in children and teenagers. The condition is annoying but not serious.

Natural treatment of nocturnal leg cramps is most effective with vitamin E. There are many studies which describe how relief was obtained by intakes of 100 i.u. with each meal, with an extra 100 i.u. dose before going to sleep. In addition, sometimes calcium supplements — preferably as dolomite (four tablets before sleep) — may help. A vitamin B_6 dosage of 10 to 25 mg often produces relief when the cramps are associated with a specific condition like pregnancy.

Night cramps in the legs should not be confused with cramps in the calves induced by walking. Calf cramps occur predominantly in males, but also affect females over forty five years old. These calf cramps are more serious, but should not be confused with pains in other muscles such as the thigh, around the knee, ankles and feet which may come on with any exertion and are often due to arthrosis in the hips, knees, ankles or feet. Both conditions need treatment, but as we shall see the natural approach to arthrosis is a separate entity.

'Growing pains'

This misnomer describes aches and pains which are popularly believed to be associated with the growing process. The fact is that growing does not of itself cause aches and pains although these are not uncommon in the arms and legs of growing children — particularly in the legs. Most of these pains are not due to serious disease. Once it was believed by anxious parents that such 'growing pains' were a sign of rheumatic fever. This fear may have been justified up until forty years ago; now however rheumatic fever is so rare that it can be discounted as a cause.

In most children, 'growing pains' are not due to arthritis or allied conditions. The reasons are more likely to be strain, fatigue, ill-health, badly fitting footwear or even a dislike of going to school. There are many empiric sources of such pains, and for some reason rapidly-growing children appear to suffer more, but in no way are such pains the result of growth. When swelling of the knees occurs (the so-called 'water on the knee', see p. 24) then arthritis may well be present but in the large majority of the children with 'growing pains' there is no swelling, just aches which will pass off as the child grows up.

Creaking, clicking and cracking joints

We have all experienced or seen so-called double-jointed people bending their fingers, toes and other joints to produce clicks and snapping noises. Although there is a popular belief that such people will later in life be arthritic cripples this is a fallacy. What is true is that double-jointed people who can bend their joints much further than normal people are more liable to suffer strains and sprains and so experience joint pains more than less elastic people. They can also injure their joints more readily because of their increased suppleness.

Once into their thirties and forties, many people experience cracking noises in their knees, feet, neck and shoulders which are even audible to others. These clicks, creaks and cracks usually accompany middle age and have no serious significance. Often grating movements can be felt with the hands over the knee-caps or across the back of the neck. These are not a sign of disease but associated with the fact of growing older and more mature. The occasional, solitary joint noise can be experienced at any age but it has so significance or connection with any disease.

Pins and needles

This sensation which we have all experienced, is common in the hands and arms and is a result of pressure on a nerve. It is rarely due to arthritis. The condition is usually caused by lying on one arm in deep sleep, by hanging an arm over a chair back which compresses the nerves in the armpit or by pressing a crutch up under the shoulder.

When the nerves of the wrist are compressed, the tingling sensation can be felt right up the arm. This tingling is often worse at night and can interfere with sleep. Nerve compression may also follow a fracture or dislocation of the wrist but it is also a feature of the menopause in some women. Occasionally it may be due to early rheumatoid arthritis, thyroid deficiency or some other disorder. Sensations of pins and needles which occur only occasionally in hands, arms, feet or legs and last only a short time are of no significance. If they persist, however, and are troublesome for days or weeks, they can be indicative of arthritis or some other disorders and professional help should be sought.

Pricking sensations in the bases of the thumbs where they meet the wrists are an early sign of osteoarthritis of this joint. This unpleasant but not serious affliction was neatly reported by the second witch on the heath in Shakespeare's *Macbeth:* 'By the pricking of my thumbs, something wicked this way comes'. She was right; but although osteoarthritis of the thumbs is unpleasant it is only a nuisance and should have no effect upon general health.

Stiff neck

An acute stiff neck may come on suddenly, often after sitting in a draught or after sleeping with the neck bent sideways. Treatment is simple; locally applied heat (a warm scarf or hot-water bottle) and rest are often sufficient to cure the condition in a few hours or days. Persistence of the pain may require massage, neck traction or manipulation at the hands of an experienced osteopath.

A long-standing stiff neck may be the result of an old injury or be due to osteoarthritis brought on by a hardening of the cartilaginous discs between the vertebrae of the neck. This condition usually occurs in old age but its development can start earlier even though the symptoms are slight.

Some of the more rare arthritic conditions, such as ankylosing spondylitis (see p. 34) appear much earlier in life, and predominantly amongst males. Arthritis is rarely a cause of stiffness of the neck but osteoarthritis, which is degeneration of the disc or joint, is the more likely cause in the sixth and seventh decades of life. Oddly, such old age stiffness is not usually accompanied by pain but when it is, the pain is not severe and is usually short-lived.

Bursitis

Bursitis means inflammation of a bursa or bursae. A bursa is a small flattened sac, or pouch, containing synovial fluid — a slippery lubricant required to reduce friction and absorb shocks at joints and tendons. These bursae are interposed between parts of the body that move on each other. The bursae which most commonly cause trouble are those at the elbow ('tennis elbow'), the shoulder joint, and the knee joint ('water on the knee', 'housemaid's knee').

The most frequent cause of bursitis is an injury, such as a knock or unusual pressure on the kneecap, or an excessive amount of exercise which can irritate the shoulder joint and elbow bursae (tennis elbow). 'Student's elbow' or 'drinker's elbow' may result from prolonged pressure of the elbow on desk or table. Bunions are another type of bursitis and usually result from ill-fitting shoes causing pressure on the bones of the foot. Bursitis may also occur as part of a generalized disease such as gout or arthritis. Usually however the cause is simply repeated friction and the condition improves when these pressures are reduced.

Heavy lifting, such as carrying home shopping, can cause bursitis in shoulders and elbows. The turning of wringers attached to some older-style washing machines can also lead to bursitis. Other and more rare forms of bursitis are caused by acute or chronic infection and need not concern us here. Contributing factors are an unsatisfactory diet containing inadequate protein, also overwork and lack of sleep.

Relief can be given by applying hot fomentations and resting and gently massaging the affected part. Later, start with gentle passive movement of the joint and increase it gradually until normal action of the joint is restored.

The following should be taken, all together, three times daily after meals:

4 Vitamin B_{12} tablets   0.025 mg
3 Rutin tablets   60 mg
1 Vitamin E tablet   50 mg
1 lecithin capsule   250 mg
3 calcium tablets (white)   60 mg
1 dessertspoonful brewers' yeast and powder, mixed in milk or water.

Frozen shoulder

The shoulder joint is characterized by a high degree of mobility resulting in a large range of movements. For this reason the tendons cross the joint in close proximity to a bursa which is there to act as a protective cushion beneath the bone. Any sort of inflammatory process in this area causes pain on movement and the various structures stick to each other resulting in the so-called frozen shoulder. Movement becomes impossible through stiffness rather than through pain.

The condition known as frozen shoulder may arise through arthritis of the shoulder joint but it is more likely to be due to generalized inflammation of the area around the joint known as periarthritis. Any sort of movements and manipulations (but particularly violent ones) make such joints worse by tearing the tissues that are stuck to each other. At one time this condition was common in drivers of horse-drawn vehicles. It was known as 'check-rein shoulder' and was induced when a horse who was being reined in or checked by the driver would suddenly throw its head forward, pulling the reins and tearing the driver's bursae. This type of frozen shoulder is now fairly rare because of the demise of horse-drawn vehicles but other sudden jerks upon the arms can produce similar conditions.

Frozen shoulder is best treated by simple but gentle exercises. As long as they are not too vigorous the condition is not exacerbated.

Tennis elbow (sometimes known as 'golfer's elbow')

This is a condition of the area where the muscle of the

elbow meets the bone and is characterized by that area becoming extremely painful and tender. Overzealous backstrokes on the tennis court can cause small tears in this muscle which lead to pain. The condition is often aggravated by frozen shoulder and the only treatment is to rest the affected joint.

Golfer's elbow is similar but usually affects the area on the other side of the elbow. Like tennis elbow the lesion can last for many months and treatment is similar, involving complete rest of the joint.

'Water on the knee'

The soft cushion-like bursae are present in large numbers around the knee and the one at the back is called Baker's cyst. It is connected to the knee joint and can thus function like an overflow tank when the knee becomes over-full with fluids. The condition, called water on the knee, can be a result of injury, excessive exercise, strain or of an arthritic lesion. It manifests itself as a bulge on the back of the knee and can be regarded as the body's way of reducing the fluid pressure in a knee joint by taking up the overflow.

Fibrositis

The names suggests an inflammation of the fibrous tissue under the skin and in the muscles, but although the term still enjoys popular use, there is no good evidence that the fibrous tissue is affected. To the sufferer it usually means just aches and pains across the neck, shoulders and upper back. There is no clear-cut cause of the pain but in most cases it is a referred pain (i.e. injury in one part causing pain in another) from areas in the neck and spine due to strains, minor injuries and degeneration in bone and cartilage.

Causes of fibrositis range from fatigue, prolonged bad posture, depression and anxiety, to fever, undue exertions in the garden or elsewhere, horse riding, and sports, particularly when these are undertaken after a long lay-off. The aches and crackles that are experienced round and under the shoulder blades and upper back are commonplace and unpleasant but are not indicative of any serious underlying disorder. The so-called 'fibrous nodules' are simply lumps of fat or fibrous tissue that are present but do not contribute to the pain.

Neuralgia

Neuralgia, sometimes called neuritis, is due to pressure on a nerve and is characterized by pins and needles, severe pain and possibly other sensations in the arm or leg. The commonest example is sciatica which is a pain arising from pressure of a low-back vertebra on a nerve root.

Trigeminal neuralgia is particularly painful in the cheek when even wiping the area with a towel can be agonizing because the area is so sensitive. There are reports of the condition being eased by high intakes of vitamin B_1 (50-600 mg daily). Sciatica too may respond to this treatment.

Shingles is due to inflammation of a nerve by the virus Herpes Zoster, which causes a pricking, burning sensation in the skin even before the rash, characteristic of the disease, appears.

Hand problems

Thickening of the hands occurs with age, particularly around the end joints of the fingers. The reason is that bone around the ageing cartilage thickens and strengthens. The palms also thicken in some people (men rather than women) and this condition is known as Dupuytren's contraction after the surgeon who first described it. This thickening of the tissues of the palms under the skin may lead to contraction of the fingers. Sometimes surgery is necessary to ease the condition, not because it is painful but because the function of the hand becomes impaired.

Ganglia are small, semi-solid humps that sometimes appear on the backs of the wrists. They may be unsightly but are of no consequence and do not hurt. At one time they were hit very hard with heavy books in attempts to flatten them but apart from their appearance they cause no harm. Occasionally they may be an early sign of rheumatoid arthritis but other signs are more likely to be indicative of this complaint.

Foot problems

Unfortunately such problems (more common in women than men) are often due to ill-fitting footwear. The most common cause is pointed shoes which have the effect of pushing all five toes into an area far too small for them, a condition not helped by high heels. The big toe is then pushed sideways towards the middle toe, the others are rearranged around the middle one and, of necessity, are displaced backwards. The end result is hard, painful areas that form in the skin from friction of the toes on the shoe above. As the big toe is pushed sideways its base suffers more friction against the shoe and the result is an inflamed area we call a bunion. Wearing high heels may cause friction in the so-called Achilles tendon running into the back of the heel. Sometimes this is also seen in ballet dancers who put their whole weight on one toe, but in this case gradual training allows the tendon to be thickened and strengthened.

A common complaint of the feet is swelling of the ankles due to water retention and this too is more common in women than in men. Prolonged immobility in standing or sitting positions, as in long car or aeroplane trips, often produces swollen ankles but these disappear once the person is mobile again. Persistent swelling can be associated with varicose veins, heart and kidney disease or even arthritis and hence it should be treated accordingly.

Most people often attribute mild persistent ankle swelling to poor circulation and in some respects this is true. The heart's action pumps blood out to the body tissues through the arteries, but by the time the blood is returned to the heart via the veins the pressure has dropped and this is overcome by muscular activity in the legs, a high muscular tone of the veins, and valves in the veins. These factors are very important since in one way human beings can be seen as containers of blood; when we stand erect our veins are full up to the top of the breastbone. The extra pressure required to make the blood reach the top of the head is supplied by the factors described. If veins become congested in the hands and feet, they immediately empty once the extremities are elevated above heart level. Similarly if the valves in our veins become weak they are unable to hold back the blood against gravity. The blood becomes stagnant in the dilated blood vessels and the result is varicose veins.

Backache

Backache is one of the commonest disabilities affecting human beings and is probably the most likely rheumatic disorder to cause time off work.

The spine is essentially a column of twenty-four vertebrae holding up the skull at the top and ending in a large bony bowl called the pelvis. Between the vertebrae are the cartilage discs, elastic cushions that act as shock absorbers. Around them are ligaments and capsules which contain many nerve endings which are sensitive to pressure, tearing and stretching. At the back are small joints between adjacent vertebrae and in some cases of arthritis it is these joints that are affected.

The spine is structured for stability and mobility so it has to be supple but sturdy. It also carries, through a tunnel in its centre, the spinal cord which connects the brain to the lumbar region. At the vertebrae, nerves leave the cord at different levels, some of them ending up in the limbs. Hence if these vertebrae pinch together or the cartilage cushion between them becomes displaced the pain may be felt in the back or transmitted to the limb which those particular nerves serve.

The commoner causes of low backache (i.e. lumbago) are fatigue, backstrain, overwork, bad posture at home, at work or whilst travelling, and even mild depression — a tiny ache may become more severe in the face of anxiety and worry. Ligaments are easily torn or strained by sudden exertions, particularly if weights are lifted with the spine bent, or as a result of sudden twisting movements and falls.

There are very few backaches that do not respond to rest, support, dietary measures or the treatments discussed later in this book but the time taken to obtain relief can vary from days to months. Time, rest and avoidance of strain are sometimes sufficient.

Other simple measures to relieve those with chronic backache include sleeping on a firm mattress, sometimes with a board beneath it. A sagging mattress will aggravate most low backaches and a firm support beneath the spine and legs will help considerably. Similarly a small cushion can help support the small of the back whilst sitting at home, in the office or whilst travelling and so prevent 'slouching' which contributes to back problems. Weights should be lifted by bending the knees and not the spine which should be kept straight.

Arthritic Disorders

The word arthritis literally means the inflammation of a joint or joints, rather than one specific condition. Sometimes there is also a degenerative condition as well and in this case the disease is better described as arthrosis.

Osteoarthritis (osteoarthrosis)

In this condition inflammatory changes are present in the joint for part of the time but the essential changes are degenerative and occur gradually over a longer period of time. What happens is that the cartilage pads that act as shock absorbers between the bones start ageing in the mid-twenties, losing their elasticity over the succeeding years. When the fifties and sixties are reached, some of these cartilages are narrowed to some extent and aches and pains may be noticed in the affected areas. Usually the most commonly affected are the finger-tip joints, the thumb bases at the wrist, the lower part of the back of the neck, the lower back, the big-toe joints and the knee.

During the process the bone-ends on each side of the affected cartilage may thicken and hence become stronger but they are unsightly and often they become stiff, causing aches and pains. Repeated small injuries play a part, particularly in the finger joints and big toes and the hard-working hand may show more thickening than the one that is used less and hence less prone to minor injuries. One example of the effect of repeated lesions in the development of osteoarthritis of the hand is seen in professional wicket-keepers who play regular cricket and in baseball catchers: their hands become gnarled but remain functional. The thumb bases develop a painful, annoying condition causing the hand to become square in the affected areas. The big-toe joint may also become painful due to degenerative changes since this is a weight-bearing joint that is more likely to suffer minor injuries, not least because of ill-fitting shoes.

Spinal osteoarthritis is usually associated with degenerative changes at the base of the neck and in the lower lumbar area, where it is commonly called lumbago. However although these areas almost always suffer some degeneration as the years advance they are only occasionally painful and only rarely is this severe. In most cases the condition appears as a direct result of advancing age but as we shall see the degenerative changes can be retarded by means of suitable diet and may not even appear.

Scoliosis, the sideways-bent spine, is rarely a cause of backache. When vertebrae are displaced, the dislocation is called spondylosis thesis and it causes little or no pain unless a nerve is trapped between them.

One particular type of spinal problem however is associated with the menopause. Once the ovarian secretion of female sex hormones ceases, calcium is lost from the vertebrae at a greater rate than it is replaced. The result is a lighter bone that is literally honeycombed and the condition is known as osteoporosis. Pain then becomes quite acute when the vertebrae become squashed and a crush fracture develops. The weakened bone readily becomes compressed giving rise to slight to severe pain that may necessitate bed rest. The only sure treatment is to attempt to replace the calcium lost from the bone and this is very difficult although there is a body of opinion which believes that dietary supplementation with the mineral represents the only safe, natural treatment.

Knees and hips. The most serious consequence of severely-affected osteoarthritic knees and hips is disability. A congenital abnormality or previous injuries can predispose to osteoarthritis because the bones may be out of proper alignment from a previous fracture, a dislocation, knock-knees or some other deformity and the condition is more likely to develop. Osteoarthritis rarely affects wrists, elbows and shoulders unless they have been previously injured.

Fortunately it does not cause loss of general health or shorten life. One important factor that does appear to contribute to development of osteoarthritis is overweight but even slim people are not completely immune.

Menopausal osteoarthritis. At the time of the menopause some women develop a type of osteo-arthritis that is characterized by aches in the finger tips, thumbs, knees, neck and back. Although relatively common in women in the western world it is rare in African women who tend to develop osteo-arthritis as a result of injury. No one knows why there is this difference since the cause of the menopause — lack of female sex hormones — is the same in all women. The reasons may be dietary, social, differences in mental and physical stress or simply racial. Fortunately these osteoarthritic conditions tend to disappear once the menopause is over.

Rheumatoid arthritis

Rheumatoid arthritis is an entirely different disease from osteoarthritis. It can affect people of any age from two years upwards. No one knows why it occurs in certain people and not others and there is little evidence of a hereditary connection although this may be a factor. It now seems, however, that the disease may be a consequence of a poor, unbalanced diet since there is little doubt that dietary changes in those affected can confer benefit.

Rheumatoid arthritis is primarily a disease of the covering about the joint. It is described as 'a disease of the joints characterized by morbid changes in the synovial membrane surrounding the smaller joints, cartilage and bones. It results in deformity, restricted movement of joints affected and muscular wasting.'

The disease is familiar to most of us, for we have seen all too frequently those changes involving the terminal and other finger joints. Sometimes the joints have become greatly enlarged. Some of the nodes (knobs or hard tumours) give little trouble except mentally, but that is trouble enough when one is aware of the possible progress of the disease.

Sometimes there is distortion of hands and wrists also, for although it particularly affects the smaller joints, the larger ones, including the elbows, frequently become affected. The joints are usually affected in the following order: hands, feet, wrists, ankles, knees and cervical vertebrae; but no joint is immune.

At first the inflammation attacks only the fibrous tissues around the joint, but unless the disease is arrested, the synovial membranes and articular cartilages will also become chronically inflamed. The cartilages may ultimately show excessive destruction, with the heads of the bones becoming bare. In some cases the movement of the joints causes a creaking and grating sound.

Women sufferers are more numerous; some give the ratio as three to one, some as high as five to one, and the onset in most cases occurs before forty years of age. If nothing is done to remove the causes, the joints gradually lose their flexibility, becoming enlarged, distorted and finally immovable. In other words, the bone becomes fixed to the socket by a slow, but insidious process of mineralization.

The four unpleasant symptoms of rheumatoid

arthritis are pain, swelling, tenderness and stiffness in the affected joints. These cause considerable disability and sometimes crippling deformity but often the disease settles down and only a minority of sufferers reach the completely crippled stage. Happily the spine is seldom affected and the neck only in the rare cases of severe rheumatoid arthritis.

Spondylitis (also known as ankylosing spondylitis)
Spondylitis is a chronic, progressive disease of arthritic origin which affects one or more of the vertebrae. The degenerative changes in the vertebrae are similar to those seen in rheumatoid arthritis. Ninety per cent of patients with spondylitis are males, often young men. The onset is usually gradual, beginning with mild back pains which become increasingly severe as the inflammation intensifies. Some cases are associated with the skin condition psoriasis and some with colitis. The condition sometimes appears in those suffering from German measles but it is short-lived and recovery is complete after a few days.

Rheumatic fever
Fortunately this disease is now rare in this country and the west generally but unhappily it still occurs in the poorer countries of the world. It is now recognized that rheumatic fever is associated with a prior streptococcal (bacterial) infection. Overcrowding, malnutrition and dampness all predispose to respiratory infections and thereby indirectly to rheumatic fever.

This fever often develops into rheumatic heart disease, which is a crippling of the heart's valvular action, thereby interfering with the passage of blood to and from the heart with a consequent disturbance of bodily function.

Rheumatic fever usually begins with a sore throat, tonsillitis, or scarlet fever. Cough, chill, fever, pleurisy and abdominal pains may be experienced. Severe joint pains generally follow and continue for some days.

According to *The Lancet,* investigations made in New York revealed that in a school for girls of wealthy parents, there had not been a case of rheumatic fever for ten years, whereas among poor children living near the school, there were many cases. *The British Medical Journal* found that there was a reduction in the number of cases of rheumatic fever when children ate eggs as part of their diet. Research indicated that patients had been eating too little protein food.

It would seem therefore that sound nutrition and good housing will effectively prevent most cases of rheumatic fever. Vitamin E has been found beneficial in restoring to health those whose hearts have been damaged by rheumatic heart disease following rheumatic fever, usually in their early youth. In an initial attack a dosage of 400 mg of vitamin E daily is needed, irrespective of age. In subsequent attacks, where there may be extensive injury to the heart, it is prudent to begin with 100 mg of vitamin E daily for two weeks and increase the daily dosage slowly by 20 mg every month, until 400-500 mg are being taken daily.

Lumbago, neuritis, sciatica

Lumbago is a rheumatic condition affecting the muscles of the lower part of the back known as the lumbar region. Unless cured by the proper principles, lumbago becomes more frequent and more painful — like all rheumatic complaints — as the sufferer gets older.

Neuritis is rheumatism or inflammation of the sciatic nerve, which runs down each hip joint. It is a particularly crippling and agonizing complaint. The sciatic nerve is the longest nerve in the body and runs clear down to the ankle. Lumbago and sciatica can be caused by draught, dampness or chill and, therefore, properly treated, need not become chronic. They can also arise from a displaced spinal disc or vertebra, and the services of a competent osteopath or chiropractor should be sought if the diet and vitamins suggested fail to bring relief.

Gout

The cause of gout is an excess of uric acid due to excessive production within the body or to faulty elimination through the kidneys or a mixture of both. The disease often runs in families but males are affected far more often than females, usually when past middle-age.

Gout differs from other types of arthritis in being characterized by excruciating pain. Arthritis has been compared to the pain produced by putting a cord around the toe and tightening it twice. Tighten it several times more and that is gout! The condition usually affects only one joint — mainly that of the big toe — producing a red shininess of the skin stretched tight by the swelling and inflammtion which gives an appearance not unlike that of a (very painful) tomato.

Gout often comes on in the night and may be precipitated by too much food, alcohol or even exercise. Foods high in purines and pyrimidines, which are constituents of nucleic acids, are more likely to give rise to gout because these substances form uric acid in the body. Such foods are liver, kidney, sweetbreads and yeast, so high intakes of these should be avoided. Oddly, changes in daily routine may contribute to gout which explains why the disease is more common in men on holidays or business tours away from home. The acute pain is due to the uric acid crystallizing into the joints and setting up a physical irritation. Dissolution of these crystals, or prevention of their formation, is thus the basis of treatment.

2
The Causes of
Rheumatic Ailments

Ten Causes of Rheumatism
The usual causes of rheumatism in its various forms
are as follows:

1 Excessive eating The British, European and
American eating tradition is one of excess food
consumption.

The average man or woman does not need more
than one-third to one-half of food usually eaten. A
breakfast of cereal and milk, followed by eggs or
grilled and fried vegetables, toast, tea or coffee, is
beyond the digestive capacity of everybody except
those people doing hard physical work. The average
lunch is also excessive, while an evening meal of meat,
vegetables and sweets merely adds insult to injury.
This excessive food intake creates more uric acid than
can be eliminated by the kidneys and sweat glands.

Excessive eating also increases the body weight
which contributes to extra pressure on the load-
bearing joints. People are healthier when slim and this
particularly applies to the arthritis sufferer. It is
therefore imperative that obesity is avoided in the
arthritic.

2 Too much meat and starchy food The protein foods (meat, fish, eggs or cheese) leave no waste bulk to stimulate bowel action. Instead, they leave an acid ash, which has chiefly to be eliminated through the kidneys. The kidneys are not equal to the task, and the uric acid accumulates in the blood stream, causing rheumatism.

The offending starchy foods are usually white bread, processed breakfast foods, refined cereals, polished rice, pappy biscuits and pastry — all of which are largely devitalized and demineralized. They are not desirable foods — merely causes of fermentation, congestion, constipation, acidity and rheumatism.

3 Incompatible food combinations The fermentation mentioned above is especially acute when we eat incompatible foods at the same meal, such as protein foods and concentrated starch foods.

4 Indiscriminate feeding Most of us have grown up in the evil dietetic tradition that all so-called food is good for us — that it's all 'grist for the mill'. We therefore proceed to eat anything and everything that comes our way, quite regardless of the appalling task we have set our digestive organs, our eliminatory organs and our body chemistry. Soup, meat, vegetables, messy puddings, washed down by tea or coffee — in it all goes. We may arise from such a meal with a strong sense of satisfaction, but we have set in motion all the factors which may finally create fermentation, flatulence, acidity — and — rheumatism.

5 *Processed foods* If that were not bad enough, our next meal may add to the offence by consisting of one or other of the doubtful concoctions, pleasing enough to look at no doubt, which fill the windows of the delicatessen shop.

Here we see a picturesque assortment of embalmed, preserved and demineralized products masquerading as 'food' in the form of pies, pastries, and an assortment of sausage meats, consisting of meat scraps, flour, fat and colouring, highly flavoured and seasoned — all acid-forming, all aiders and abettors of rheumatism in one or other of its forms.

6 *Condiments* are a further potent contribution to an acid blood-stream.

7 *Sugar* also stands indicted for its acid-forming qualities. To quote from *Your Diet in Health and Disease* by Harry Benjamin:

All refined sugar is useless, needless, and harmful, as it requires a great deal of oxygen for its combustion in the tissues and prevents the oxygen being used for other and more important purposes.

In addition, the heat it generates, not being required for the work of the body generally, is so much waste fuel, and the end products of its combustion being excessively acid, they require a proportionately large amount of mineral salts, which the body can ill afford, for their neutralization. . .

8 *Devitalized and demineralized foods* White bread, refined breakfast foods, biscuits, polished rice, etc. are

all acid-forming — all stepping stones to rheumatic ailments.

9 *Excessive tea and coffee drinking* Both are acid-forming. Incidentally, wine is notorious for its formation of acidity.

10 *A diet woefully deficient in vitamin A, the B complex vitamins, vitamins C, D and E* The B complex vitamins and vitamin C are particularly important for the prevention, and the relief, of rheumatism.

Broadly these are the ten sins of commission which between them, give rise to an acid blood-stream and finally rheumatism in one of its forms.

These sins of commission are aggravated by those who eat inadequately of the foods that alkalize the blood and give it its proper chemical balance — such foods as fresh fruits and salad vegetables, and to a lesser extent dried and stewed fruits and cooked vegetables (see p. 68).

Sir W. Arbuthnot Lane, one of Britain's greatest surgeons and nutritional authorities, wrote:

There is no longer any doubt that all forms of rheumatism are due to disturbance of the acid-alkaline balance, and that this condition arises from faults in nutrition. Clinical experience has now amply proved that the physical factors which predispose some people to rheumatism can only be successfully countered by a diet which puts all its emphasis upon alkaline-forming foods.

Dr Adrian Vander, a European authority upon modern medical science, has written in his book

Rheumatism and Gout:
> The whole group of rheumatic illnesses is nothing but the result of an abnormal, i.e. diseased, alteration in the composition of the bodily fluids. . . This has its origin in the first place in the acidification of the body (especially with uric acid and oxalic acid).

Diet

The energy constituents of the diet, although falling into the basic categories of carbohydrates, fats and protein, also contribute to the acidity or alkalinity of the body depending upon how they ultimately break down. Hence foods may be acid-forming or alkaline-forming or in some cases neither. The categories into which each foodstuff falls are now well established and tables have been published indicating whether the food gives excess acid or excess base (alkali). There is evidence that a diet consisting mainly of acid-forming foods is more likely to give rise to arthritic conditions than one with a preponderance of alkali-forming foods. Hence we may regard acid-forming foods as one cause of rheumatism and so avoid them in the dietary treatment of the complaint.

Acidity: parent of disease
The acid-forming foods are:

meat	biscuits
fish	alcoholic liquors
poultry	macaroni and spaghetti
oysters	sugar
cheese	jam

eggs	fried foods
bread	strong tea
flour	coffee
pastry	common salt
pies	sauces
rice	condiments
confectionery	pickles
'soft' drinks	condensed milk
cakes	pre-cooked and processed cereals

If you suffer from rheumatism, check over the list and you will probably see that these are the foods which have made up the bulk of your diet for most of your life. They are acid-forming and acidity is often the parent of rheumatism.

You may reply that the foods listed constitute the diet of 95 per cent of the people of this country, and that many people seem to be able to eat this acid-forming food year after year without getting rheumatism. Yet nobody knows exactly how far these apparently immune people have progressed, unbeknown to themselves, towards a rheumatic condition.

It does not follow, of course, that everybody who eats the acid-forming foods we have listed will contract rheumatism. But one thing is certain: practically every human being who persists with an acid-forming diet, unleavened with a preponderance of alkaline-forming fruits and vegetables, will very likely eventually fall victim to rheumatism, kidney disease, heart disease, high blood-pressure, or chronic ill-health.

Four sources of acidity

Dr Howard Hay has stated that the four known sources of acid-formation in the body, according to modern medical science, are as follows:

(a) The use of too much of the concentrated foods: meats, eggs, fish, cheese, dried peas, beans, lentils, nuts, bread and all grain foods.

(b) The free use of those foods from which the normal alkalines are lost as in processed starches, sugar and sweets of all kinds, white bread, pastries, refined breakfast cereals, sugars, synthetic syrups, candies.

(c) The incompatible mixing of foods of all kinds, e.g. the starches or sugars with either the acid fruits or the protein foods.

(d) The retention of food residues in the large bowel beyond the twenty-four hours that mark the outside limit of safety.

The value of acid fruits

Dr N. W. Walker, a doctor of science, points out that lemon juice and grapefruit juice aid in the removal or dissolving of minerals which have formed deposits in the cartilage of the joints (as in arthritis) as the result of excessive consumption of acid-forming foods.

As a general rule, acid fruits are not acid forming; they neutralize body acids. But such fruits may aggravate the condition of sufferers from acute arthritis and rheumatism, as these people's digestive processes may not be able to deal with the juices and render them alkaline.

Other useful alkalizers for correcting excess acidity are alfalfa and such vegetables as celery, watercress, parsley, mint and horseradish. Alfalfa tablets, also vegetable tablets (containing the five above-mentioned vegetables, together with birch — all valuable for acidity) are available.

Gout and diet

There is no doubt that gout is precipitated by rich foods and drink. The reason is not hard to find. Rich foods, which are usually of animal origin, by the very nature of their structure contribute large intakes of what are known as purines and pyrimidines to the diet. These substances are present in the ribonucleic and deoxyribonucleic acids that are important cell constituents, particularly in liver, kidney, heart and other offal foods. These acids perform essential lifegiving functions in the living animal but they contribute nothing to the diet when the animal is eaten. What happens to them after absorption from the digestive system is that the body, particularly the liver, metabolizes them to other substances which are eventually excreted.

The central metabolite in this system is uric acid which the body is usually able to handle effectively on its way to excretion. When excessive amounts of purines and pyrimidines are eaten, however, too much uric acid is produced. The body cannot get rid of it and the uric acid crystallizes into the joints, causing the excruciating pain associated with gout. Purines and pyrimidines are not confined to animal foods and it must be remembered that yeast is a rich source of these compounds. Hence, too much yeast can also precipitate gout in susceptible people.

The Contribution of Stress

During the 1950s, animal experiments established beyond doubt that stress situations of both the physical and mental kinds increased their requirements of the vitamin B complex and vitamin C. Confirmation that human beings also required more of these vitamins during periods of stress soon followed, notably in the case of astronauts. These people, who in the early days of space flight were fed diets based on daily allowances of vitamins for earthbound individuals, all were found to be biochemically deficient in vitamins when they returned to earth. The deficiencies were associated with the stress of space take-off and flight, and supplementation with extra vitamins in subsequent flights solved the problem.

In a similar fashion stress can cause certain diseases such as arthritis, and lack of the vitamin B complex and vitamin C in particular are a feature of the complaint. The anti-stress hormones produced in the adrenal cortex depend upon these vitamins for adequate synthesis. Lack of vitamins may reduce the ability of the gland to produce these hormones and the end-result is a stress-related disease like arthritis. This explains why treatment with certain vitamins can often relieve the symptoms of arthritis and these are discussed in more detail later in the book (see p. 69-75).

Hence one cause of arthritis can be a long-term deficiency of certain vitamins induced by poor diet or by mental stress. In the case of athletes stress is both physical (excessive exercise) and mental (that of competition). The ultimate result is a high incidence of arthritic and related diseases in these individuals.

The progress of arthritis is illustrated in the following chart which summarizes the various factors that can contribute to the disease.

Fig. 1. The Progress of Arthritis

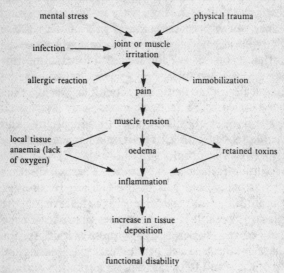

Causes Due to the Weather

As for the weather causing rheumatism — this has no basis in fact. If it were true, then people of the cold, wet countries, such as the British Isles, Northern Europe and Russia would be martyrs to rheumatism. The fact is that the people of these countries do not suffer any more from this ailment than other people do. Indeed, some authorities say that the incidence of rheumatism is more general in Australia than in the European countries named. Undoubtedly the rheumatic sufferer reacts to sudden changes in the weather, but this is because his or her condition is affected by the weather. This is very different from saying that the rheumatism was caused by the weather in the first place.

Damp, chilly weather does, however, depress the circulation and cold draughts can lower one's resistance by causing constriction of the blood vessels. This interferes with the elimination of waste products from the muscles and surrounding areas, thereby setting up an inflammatory condition conducive to fibrosis. To take drugs is futile because local treatment, i.e. steam baths, or hot and cold compresses are needed, as discussed later (p. 102-5). A faulty diet can be a contributing factor because it will load the body with toxic substances, so that an attack of fibrositis will be more severe and of longer duration than if the body's powers of resistance were higher.

The ills of winter are partly due to the fact that we are denied the benefit of summer's perspiration, and thus accumulate additional poisons in the system which lower our resistance to epidemics. In addition, in winter we eat more of the heating, acid-forming foods, and eat less of the vitalizing fruits and salad vegetables.

Rheumatism is often the result of an accumulation of acidity in the muscles or joints. By building up the alkalinity of the blood stream and by adequate and regular elimination, without the assistance of purgative medicines, the severity of attacks may be lessened and in many cases averted.

Rheumatism Can Be Arrested

Dr Howard Hay, when asked 'What is rheumatism? How can it be corrected?' gave the following answer:

Rheumatism is a general name for all sorts of painful inflammation about the joints and muscles, some of which are called arthritis, some simple rheumatism, acute, sub-acute, and chronic, some synovitis or water in the joint, and no doubt much neuritis passes as rheumatism.

All these things are merely deposits of salts representing waste matter, or toxic-serum or lymph in the case of the watery infiltrations. These are to be corrected by neutralizing the acidity and eliminating the waste, though it may be a slow process.

In the case of arthritis, there are salts such as urates that are actually outside the circulation, deposited in the free joint cavity and not absorbable, usually so constituting a permanent crippling to just this extent.

All forms are easily arrested, and all but arthritis recover easily and quickly under drastic detoxication and corrected diet.

3

Effects of
Orthodox Therapies

The orthodox approach to the problem of rheumatism in its several forms consists of medicines, pain-killing drugs, vaccines and gold injections, with embrocations, liniments and creams to rub in.

Clement Jeffrey, in his book *Rheumatism,* wrote:

While writing this book I have eagerly examined the best authorities for any guidance which I could give to the reader in the use of medicines for rheumatism; but drugs are a failure.

I have mentioned that asprrin can give relief from pain, but it has the disadvantage of disturbing the digestion and producing an unnatural sweat.

There can be little doubt that this perspiration is an attempt on the part of Nature to expel the aspirin from the system.

Dr Buckley states in his book on arthritis, fibrositis and gout that the number of drugs which have been tried in rheumatic diseases is legion. This, he adds, is a testimony to their general futility.

Dr Copeman (in his *Short History of Gout and Rheumatic Diseases,* University of California Press, 1964) is even more outspoken. 'Drugs,' he states, 'are comparatively useless in this disease except with the object of dulling pain and producing sleep.'

Let us look now at some of the conventional drug therapies and examine how they might affect you.

Aspirin

Aspirin is still the number one drug used in treating arthritic disorders but the doses needed are far in excess of the one or two tablets taken for the occasional headache or cold. A daily intake of 3.6 grams of aspirin (i.e. 12 tablets) or more is the commonly recommended dose for active rheumatoid arthritis. Unfortunately only doses below 2.4 grams of aspirin daily have few side effects so anyone on the higher dose for any length of time is almost guaranteed to suffer from adverse reactions. These include gastrointestinal discomfort, ulceration and gastric bleeding leading to serious loss of blood in some people. Nausea is common and the hearing may be affected resulting in tinnitus (ringing in the ears) and deafness. Vertigo (a sense of loss in balance) is not unusual with high intakes of aspirin and there may even be mental confusion. The person may become hypersensitive so that water retention, bronchial troubles such as asthma and skin rashes will appear. More rarely blood diseases, particularly those due to an inability to make platelets (small white blood-cells) develop. There is no treatment for these side effects apart from stopping taking the drug, and in some people they are irreversible.

However, aspirin has more insidious effects including destruction and overexcretion of vitamin C and pantothenic acid, a member of the vitamin B complex.

What is tragic is that both of these vitamins play essential roles both in reducing the inflammation of arthritis and in the body's own mechanisms for overcoming the illness. When we consider that the adverse effect of aspirin on vitamin C in the body has been known since 1936 it is sad that the vitamin is never prescribed with the drug.

In the presence of aspirin, vitamin C excretion in the urine increases and in addition actual destruction of the vitamin takes place. What was apparent from the many experiments that have taken place is that vitamin C, when taken with the drug, can actually reduce some of the side effects. Thus the aspirin is better absorbed and its adverse effect of inducing stomach bleeding is reduced dramatically. Taking vitamin C with aspirin therefore has these benefits and also replaces the vitamin lost through destruction and excretion. A typical regime would be 100 mg vitamin C taken at the same time with every two aspirin tablets after meals.

Pantothenic acid should be taken in a daily dose of 100 mg to replace that destroyed by aspirin.

Phenylbutazone
Phenylbutazone is another drug widely used in treating arthritic disease, in particular gout and ankylosing spondylitis. Like aspirin it induces bleeding in the stomach. It is not known if vitamin C will reduce this effect but it is still a wise precaution to supplement with the vitamin when taking the drug.

Phenylbutazone has two rare and dangerous adverse effects. It causes water retention and in some patients this is serious enough to precipitate heart failure.

Another serious side effect is blood disease where the bone marrow ceases to produce red and white blood-cells. This results in serious anaemia and the lack of white blood-cells will reduce the natural resistance to disease and so lay the patient wide open to infection.

Side effects occur in 20-40 per cent of patients taking phenylbutazone and these can be serious enough to cause withdrawal of the drug in 10-15 per cent. They include gastrointestinal discomfort, ulceration, bleeding, nausea, water retention, high blood-pressure, vertigo and insomnia. Skin rashes, goitre, fatal blood diseases and hepatitis are rarer but more serious. When injected the drug may cause the formation of abscesses and nerve damage.

Other comparable drugs, known as a group as non-steroidal anti-inflammatories, are Indomethacin, Naproxen, Fenbufen, Ibuprofen, Sulindac, Mefenamic Acid and many other variants. All have side effects similar to phenylbutazone and in addition may induce allergic disorders, including asthma, and liver and kidney impairment.

Cortisone and ACTH

Cortisone is a naturally-occuring hormone elaborated by the adrenal cortex. ACTH is another hormone produced in the gland known as the pituitary. Normally the pituitary gland controls the synthesis of cortisone in the body. Its action therefore is to stimulate the adrenal cortex to produce cortisone, so whether given as this or as ACTH the end result is the same — increased levels of cortisone in the body.

Cortisone and ACTH were originally hailed as 'wonder drugs' for the treatment of rheumatoid arthritis. So many wonder drugs are dramatically announced, only to result in their great promise being tragically disappointing, that any new one must be regarded with reservation until the claims made for it are definitely proved by extensive clinical experience.

Just what is ACTH? Where does it come from? How is it prepared? How does it act?

The letters ACTH stand for 'adrenocorticotrophic hormone'. For the preparation of ACTH, pituitary glands from slaughtered animals are used, preferably pigs' glands, which have been found to yield the highest percentage of ACTH per weight of gland. Sheep and oxen glands, in that order, are also used. The glands, taken from the skulls as soon after death as possible, are put into acetone to preserve them. (It takes 1,500-1,800 pig pituitary glands to make up 1 lb weight.) Later, in the laboratory, the glands are minced, and the minced matter extracted and purified to give a crude ACTH fraction. This, further purified to a whitish powder, is only a minute percentage of the original gland matter, indicating that there is a very definite limit to the amount of ACTH which can be made available.

Side effects of cortisone and ACTH

As soon as cortisone came to public notice, mainly as a healing agent for arthritis sufferers, thousands were given new hope, if only because of the claims made for the drug overseas. The same sort of thing happened with ACTH. But the important point to remember is that neither ACTH nor cortisone is a cure. They do not kill germs, nor do they remove toxins. They merely act as a shield between whatever is causing the illness, and the patient. *Provided the administration of the drug is kept up.*

ACTH has been shown to act most effectively — but, unfortunately, most transiently — on sufferers from rheumatoid arthritis. They lose their pain, swelling and depression — *until the relapse that comes so often and so swiftly after a matter of hours.*

The Mayo Clinic cites the case of a woman — a hopeless polyarthritis cripple with no movement at all — who was transformed into a comfortable, happy person without pain at the time of discharge from hospital. Two weeks later she returned in a wheel-chair, her depression and polyarthritis condition much worse than before.

But graver side effects are coming to light. For instance, Dr Gregory Schwartzman, of the Mount Sinai Hospital, New York, has shown that susceptibility to poliomyelitis is enhanced by the use of ACTH and cortisones. Other doctors believe that, administered unwisely, the hormone drugs may have a detrimental effect on patients' mental health.

As much as thirty years ago, Lord Horder, physician to King George VI in London, issued this warning: 'Cortisone is giving us and will give us more rheumatic patients left at the stage where their disabilities require treatment, than before they had cortisone.'

A leading Sydney medical practitioner writing in the *Sydney Sunday Telegraph* said:

As the months slip by, patients and doctors are being rapidly disillusioned about the new 'wonder drugs', ACTH and cortisone.

These remedies have received great publicity,

and as a result of this, many sick people are rushed into hospital for a great variety of conditions and diseases in order that these new drugs may be given a trial. . . The relatives are also anxious that everything that can be done should be done. . . The type and pattern of the response of the human body to these substances is now becoming fairly clear. . . Doctors are beginning to realize that they now suppress symptoms of various diseases, but do not have the slightest effect on the underlying cause. . . If the trouble is not serious, and is of short duration, cortisone makes the symptoms disappear until the disease runs its course. . . When treatment is stopped the patient feels and remains well. But if, on the other hand, the cause of the disease persists and the treatment is stopped symptoms return overnight, frequently with greater severity than before the treatment began. . . It does not do to take the use of these drugs too lightly. . . Sometimes death occurs while they are still under the influence of them, and gross psychological disturbances have been reported. This is a serious complication of their use. . . The present position is that the wonder has gone out of the 'wonder drugs', and we are left with a potent, but tricky remedy with which to fight symptoms, but not to cure disease.

Injurious effects of cortisone
In an article in the *Journal of the American Medical Association*, Paul H. Curtiss, Jr, M.D., William S. Clark, M.D., and Charles H. Herndon, M.D., describe four male patients with rheumatoid arthritis

'in whom severe compression fractures of the vertebrae have developed during the administration of cortisone or corticotropin or both'.

The authors go on to say, 'Although demineralization of the skeleton is a recognized complication of cortisone therapy, these cases have prompted the authors to emphasize the importance of possible pathological fractures when prolonged treatment of this nature is used.' In other words, it is quite well known among physicians that giving cortisone may result in drawing the minerals out of the bones of patients so that the bones fracture or break.

In one of the cases described, a fifty-seven-year-old man was given cortisone and corticotropin for arthritis. After six months on cortisone, the doctors stopped giving it and the patient's temperature shot up. So they gave him corticotropin. When he came back to the hospital about two years later (we assume he had been taking the drugs all this time) he had the 'moon face' and the 'buffalo hump' that seem to accompany long dosage with cortisone, also a haemorrhaging disorder of his skin. An x-ray showed that there was 'partial collapse' of five vertebrae.

A sixty-seven-year-old patient who had also been taking cortisone for arthritis had a fracture of one vertebra and 'extensive generalized demineralization' of all the vertebrae. The third patient was a nine-year-old boy suffering from arthritis. In this case, too, there were fractures and 'demineralization' of the vertebrae. The fourth case was that of a sixty-five-year-old man whose x-rays showed fractures of two vertebrae and two ribs, and osteoporosis (a softening of the bone) in his thigh bones. The authors explain that such conditions are apparently the result of excessive loss of calcium, phosphorus and nitrogen, presumably caused by the cortisone.

Medical journal's warning
Articles from the *Journal of the American Medical Association* the *Cambria County Medical Society Bulletin,* the *British Medical Journal, The Lancet,* and the *International Medical Digest,* pointed out that:

1 Cortisone paralyzes the body's natural defences against infection.
2 Cortisone may produce harmful symptoms in cases of tuberculosis, schizophrenia, diabetes and peptic ulcer.
3 Cortisone masks the symptoms by which doctors recognize the progress of diseases in patients, so that the disease may go on its deadly way while the patient feels good enough to go back to work. If the cortisone is withdrawn, symptoms will probably return and may be even worse. Or the patient may contract some infectious disease since his defences against infection have been lowered.

An article by Dr Walter C. Alvarez in his column *Your Health,* indicates that autopsies of many patients who had taken cortisone (for only five days in some cases) showed atrophy of the adrenal glands. What may we suppose has become of these glands by the time the patient has taken cortisone over a period of several years? There seems to be little chance that they could be coaxed back to normal functioning again. In addition, administration of cortisone may bring about severe reactions on such varied parts of the body as the skin, kidneys, blood, sex organs, hair, stomach, mind and personality, nerves, heart and blood vessels.

The most obvious side effect noticeable to the patient on steroids is the 'Cushing syndrome' characterized by moon face, stretch marks (striae) and acne. All are reversible on withdrawal of treatment but it is essential that this is tapered to prevent adrenal insufficiency. Nowadays cortisone is rarely used. It has been replaced by synthetic hormones that are alleged to have less side effects. They are also more potent weight for weight. Unfortunately earlier hopes have not been realized and drugs such as Prednisone, and Prednisolone that are widely used in arthritic complaints still exhibit serious side effects (see cortisone) during long-term use. These drugs, called corticosteroids, are not usually given to children since they prevent growth. In severe cases, corticosteroids may be injected directly into the affected joint which tends to produce fewer side effects than when given orally.

Gold Injections

Gold injections are considered to be disease-specific in that they are said to affect the disease process in rheumatoid arthritis and related conditions but do not affect other types of inflammatory arthritis. They differ from other anti-inflammatory drugs in a number of ways: there is no immediate response but a period of treatment of four to six months may be necessary to feel the benefit. They improve the signs and symptoms of joint disease but in addition they reduce nodule formation. Gold injections tend to be used where treatment with other anti-inflammatories has failed so they should be regarded as the ultimate therapy.

One disadvantage of gold is that it must be injected into the muscle — it cannot be taken orally. Treatment always ceases when blood diseases or kidney complaints appear. Rashes are common and their appearance always results in discontinuation of the therapy.

Side effects of gold (given as sodium aurothiomalate) are severe in 5 per cent of patients, sometimes resulting in death. They include mouth ulcers, skin reactions, water retention, protein in the urine (indicating kidney damage), blood diseases, colitis, nerve complaints and lung problems.

Penicillamine

Penicillamine and related drugs are also sometimes used in rheumatoid arthritis where there are troublesome features such as inflamed blood vessels and in those patients suffering from excessive doses of corticosteroids. When successful, penicillamine can allow a striking reduction in requirements of these steroids and other drugs. Children tend to be treated by penicillamine or gold because corticosteroids can affect their growth.

Penicillamine does however have its full complement of side effects that include allergic reactions, nausea, loss of appetite, taste loss, mouth ulcers, muscle weakness and rashes. Skin haemorrhage, water retention, protein in the urine, blood problems and fever may also occur.

Drugs To Treat Gout

Indomethacin, Naproxen and Phenylbutazone are all used to treat acute attacks of gout. Adverse effects of these drugs have been discussed on p. 53-4. In addition, however, Allopurinol, Colchicine and Probenecid are all specific for treating gout.

Allopurinol commonly causes skin rashes, sometimes with fever and this is enough to warrant discontinuation of the product. Drowsiness and gastro-intestinal disturbances may also occur. More rarely malaise, headache, vertigo, loss of taste, high blood-pressure, loss of hair and hepatitis appear.

Colchicine gives rise to nausea, vomiting, abdominal pain, diarrhoea, gastrointestinal haemorrhage, skin rashes and kidney damage. Occasionally inflammation of the nerves, alopecia and blood diseases result.

Probenecid has infrequent side effects but they include nausea, vomiting, frequency in passing urine, headaches, hot flushes, dizziness and skin rashes. Allergic reactions, kidney disease, liver impairment and aplastic anaemia (non-production of red blood-cells) do occur, but only rarely.

4

Natural Remedial Principles

In the meantime, many people in all parts of the world have proved that the following principles, consistently and resolutely followed month after month, will in time improve the condition of rheumatoid arthritis or osteoarthritis. (In the case of elderly people, with a long-standing condition of rheumatoid arthritis, the principles cannot be expected to be as effective a remedy, but they will greatly relieve the condition and vastly improve general health.) The same principles will correct the simpler forms of rheumatism, such as fibrositis, in a matter of months.

Dietary Principles

The first step towards curing rheumatism is to *stop causing it*, that is the dead, devitalized acid-forming foods (listed earlier on p. 43-4) must form no part of your daily diet.

If your rheumatic condition is bad, cut down on meat for a while. If it is not so bad take a little meat with compatible food combinations. Cut down on bread to two slices of wholemeal bread daily. Dispense with highly-refined breakfast cereals altogether. Substitute wheatgerm, milk and fruit.

Diluted fruit juices rich in vitamin C should be taken daily — orange, lemon, grapefruit, pineapple or apple juice. Reject the fallacy that acid fruits create acidity — they do just the opposite. Their reaction in the blood is 100 per cent alkaline. All acid fruits are wonderful in alkalizing the blood, except — as already stated — in cases of acute arthritis and rheumatism.

Remember, the benefit obtained depends on just one factor: how well you succeed in changing an acid, poisoned, unhealthy blood stream into a blood stream with the proper acid-alkaline balance, free from poisonous debris, and carrying a normal blood supply to every organ, every muscle, every nerve in your body.

In all your eating adopt these essential principles; first, make sure your daily diet consists of about three-quarters of alkaline-forming foods, and only about one-quarter of the acid-forming foods; and second, make sure that your diet is supplemented with the vitamins mentioned later (see p. 78).

Raw Food

Tests carried out by British medical men on people suffering with all types of rheumatic ailments and reported in the *Proceedings of the Royal Society of Medicine* (Vol. 30) showed that great benefit was obtained by a diet of all-raw food. At no time during the period the diet was in operation was any salt added to the food. We reproduce below a sample day's menu:

Breakfast Apple porridge made of grated apple, soaked raw oatmeal, grated nuts, cream, fresh orange, tea with milk or cream (no sugar).

Mid-morning Tomato pureé with lemon.

Dinner Salad of lettuce, cabbage, tomato, root vegetables, salad dressing with oil, mixed fruit salad with cream.

Tea Dried fruits, nuts and tea with milk or cream.

Supper Fruit porridge, prune, apricot or apple, salad dish with dressing.

Bedtime Lemon and orange juice with hot water.

The dried fruits and raw oatmeal were soaked in water, the vegetables were shredded and the nuts were crushed or whole. All food was prepared fresh for every meal and was served attractively.

All of the patients lost weight on the diet during the first week, but those who continued in the following weeks lost much less, and in every case except very obese patients, weight was properly maintained on the diet. For the obese patients the loss of weight was very helpful, as being overweight adds greatly to the problems of being arthritic.

Practically all the patients showed a great improvement after having been on the all-raw food diet.

The Hay Diet

The Hay Diet was developed by Dr William Howard Hay some sixty years ago after his research and observations led him to believe that highly refined carbohydrates and processed foods were the major cause of many Western diseases, including arthritis. He advised reducing the intake of meat, fat, sugar, salt and greatly increasing fibre intake by replacing these foods with fresh fruit, fresh vegetables, potatoes and wholewheat bread. His rationale was simple: disease has one underlying cause, that of incorrect chemistry of the body induced by bad diet. One consequence is a build up of toxins — acids that the body cannot get rid of — and it is these that are the basis of disease.

The Hay Diet is based on five simple rules:

1 Starches and sugars should not be eaten with proteins and acid fruits at the same meal.

2 Vegetables, salads and fruits should be the major constituents of the diet.

3 Proteins, starches and fats should be eaten only in small quantities at a time.

4 Only wholegrain and unrefined foods should be eaten since these contain complex carbohydrates (such as starch) that are more beneficial than sugars. Refined foods contain more sugar and less starches and so are to be avoided.

5 There should be at least four hours between meals of different constituents.

Concentrated proteins are found in meat, fish, cheese and poultry. Concentrated carbohydrates are a feature of wholegrains, bread, cereals and potatoes. Each type of food contains a certain small proportion of the other type but the important point is to separate the foods predominant in either protein or carbohydrate into distinct meals.

Dr Howard Hay on Arthritis

Dr Howard Hay has written in *Some Human Ailments:*

There is no such thing as an incurable case of arthritis, although damage done to the joints previously by years of arthritis may never be fully corrected. The process, however, can be halted, and a great deal of improvement enjoyed in every case. There are salts such as urates (any salt of uric acid) that are actually outside the circulation, deposited in the free joint cavity, and not usually absorbable, and so constituting a permanent crippling to just this extent.

I would not touch starch or sugar in any form, but would live entirely on cooked vegetables, raw vegetable salads, fresh fruit and milk or buttermilk and cheese. In addition, I would suggest that you get a preparation of wheatgerm and take a tablespoonful of this three times a day with honey. . .

It is not unusual to have a marked aggravation of the arthritis after you first begin changing the body's chemistry, and this is caused not by anything you are eating, but by chemicals already stored in your body that are still being precipitated. Go on in this way for a number of weeks, and you will find the condition arrested, for the pain is less and the attacks of acute arthritis less frequent and less severe.

The Alkaline-forming Foods

We have seen already that the acid-forming foods are more liable to induce the arthritic state and hence are to be avoided. In contrast, the alkaline-forming foods (most fruit and vegetables) will neutralize the acid toxins believed to be a factor in the development of the disease.

So, the healthful alkaline-forming foods are:

lemons	raspberries
oranges	blackberries
lettuce	papaws
carrots	raisins
tomatoes	pineapple
green beans	apples
grapefruit	celery
peaches	bananas
grapes	parsley
nectarines	peas (green)
cherries	apricots
strawberries	dried fruits
watercress	dates
mint	horseradish

Spinach and rhubarb should only be eaten in small amounts because their high oxalic acid content neutralizes some of the calcium in the blood stream. Their asset, however, is that they are rich in iron and other minerals.

Make a practice of having for breakfast nothing except a glass of milk and three dessertspoonsful of wheatgerm with some raisins and honey for added energy. And have a large greenleaf salad every day.

Avoid Salt

A diet low in salt (preferably free from salt altogether) is most helpful in treating all forms of rheumatism. Try leaving the salt-cellar off the table and begin omitting salt from the dishes you prepare. After a time you will discover that food is more palatable when you can taste its natural flavour instead of a heavy impregnation with salt.

Most food is adequately salted by nature. The salt we add is excessive. Salt often silts up the veins and arteries, stiffens the joints and makes them painful, intensifies migraine headaches, aggravates catarrh and eczema, raises blood pressure to dangerous heights, injures the health in other ways and makes us prematurely old and decrepit.

Kelp granules sprinkled on food, will add savour and also supply essential 'trace' elements.

Sugar and Arthritis

According to a book written by Melvin Page, entitled *Degeneration — Regeneration*, an imbalance in the calcium-phosphorus ratio of the blood can bring about an arthritic condition. Dr Page found in his researches that refined white sugar, which neutralizes calcium in the blood stream, is the principal factor in upsetting the normal calcium-phosphorus balance. So refined cane sugar should be eliminated from the diet of anyone who suffers with rheumatism and arthritis.

Rheumatism and Vitamin C Deficiency

W. J. McCormick, M.D., of Toronto, Canada, writing in the *Journal of Applied Nutrition*, considers that rheumatism and arthritis are not degenerative diseases resulting from a process of ageing, but arise basically from malnutrition, and more particularly from a lack of vitamin C. He also associates rheumatism and arthritis with a form of scurvy.

Scurvy is a nutritional disorder caused by a deficiency of vitamin C. It is characterized by spongy, bleeding gums, loosening of the teeth, haemorrhages from mucous membranes, anaemia, painful hardening of the muscles, and thickening of the bones.

Dr McCormick points out that research workers found by animal experiments that a prolonged lack of vitamin C in the diet produced functional impairment and anatomical changes in the joints, typical of rheumatism and arthritis.

It is interesting to note that ailments which indicate forms of scurvy, namely; spongy gums (pyorrhoea), loosening of the teeth, anaemia, painful hardening of the muscles and bone lesions, all respond to vitamin C. It is noteworthy, too, that vitamin C is the most vulnerable of all vitamins. It is destroyed when vegetables become stale; it is lost by the heat of cooking, and leaches away in cooking water. Baking soda destroys it. We destroy 25 mg of vitamin C every time we smoke a cigarette. People who take aspirin and other drugs lose vitamin C rapidly.

When public surveys are conducted in the USA they reveal a general vitamin C deficiency. Thus, the US Department of Agriculture in a survey of 6,000 households found that 25 per cent were not obtaining the bare minimum requirements of 75 mg daily, i.e. scarcely enough to prevent scurvy.

It is more than probable that a serious vitamin C deficiency also exists in Europe and Australia and that it arises from malnutrition, incorrect methods of feeding and the excessive use of tobacco and drugs. One of the results of this deficiency of vitamin C could well be the prevalence of rheumatism and arthritis and associated ailments.

The Value of the Flavonoids

It is now known that vitamin C functions best when taken with the flavonoids (vitamin P). Maximum benefits are obtained (according to research workers as reported in *The Journal of American Geriatrics*) by taking these two vitamins together.

The research was conducted in America by a team of highly-qualified and practical physicians. Their patients numbered 59: 17 with osteoarthritis and 42 with rheumatoid arthritis. Some had suffered over a period of seven years.

The preparation used in the tests was vitamin C with hesperidin (one of the flavonoids). The dosage used was 600 mg daily of both vitamin C and hesperidin and very good results were achieved in all the cases mentioned.

Rutin, another flavonoid, gives good results with vitamin C, and hesperidin and rutin tablets are available (both with vitamin C).

The Role of the B Complex Vitamins

Another important factor in building up the body's health to conquer rheumatism is to see that you have sufficient of the vitamin B complex group. There are about twelve vitamins in this group, most of them of fundamental importance to good health.

With rheumatism, the nerves and nerve sheaths in the affected part become inflamed due to being saturated with acidity. The B complex vitamins are essential to a healthy nervous system. With a sound diet and the B complex vitamins, the painful characteristics of rheumatism usually disappear gradually.

The main sources of the B complex vitamins are brewer's yeast, wheatgerm, crude molasses, wholemeal, unpolished rice, and liver. Milk and greenleaf vegetables contain a little. B complex tablets are also available.

As a general principle of good health, everybody should have three to four dessertspoonfuls of wheatgerm for breakfast instead of processed cereals. Take it with plenty of milk, and some honey and raisins, which add both sweetening and energy. In addition, be sure to take one B complex vitamin tablet after each meal. Both the wheatgerm — which contains ten of the vitamin B group — and the B complex vitamin tablets should become a regular part of your diet for the rest of your days.

It is also advisable to take added vitamin B_1 — one 10 mg B_1 tablet after each meal will rob arthritis of some of its pain, for this vitamin possesses analgesic as well as nutritive properties.

In his important work *Arthritis — A Vitamin Deficiency Disease* E. C. Barton-Wright strongly recommends pantothenic acid (calcium pantothenate) — a part of the B vitamin — for osteoarthritis; and pantothenic acid and royal jelly for rheumatoid arthritis.

Sun Baths and Vitamin D

Rheumatic and arthritic sufferers are advised by Dr Adrian Vander to take sun baths whenever possible because of their beneficial influence. Sun baths make the skin less sensitive to weather changes and improve the circulation of the blood near the skin surface. Exposure to the sun must be moderate at first to enable the skin to build up its defensive pigment, otherwise the skin may be badly burned.

The ultra-violet rays in sunlight cause the oil glands of the skin to create a provitamin, which is converted by the body into vitamin D and then absorbed by the blood stream.

During the winter months, owing to the sun's lower altitude and bad weather, sunlight is weak and intermittent and fewer ultra-violet rays reach the earth. Vitamin D should then be taken in capsule form to make good this deficiency. A vitamin D capsule taken twice daily after meals will do this, in conjunction with one vitamin A tablet daily — not to exceed 2,500 i.u.s.

Vitamin D is essential for healthy bones and teeth. It also releases energy within the body and helps to maintain normal heart action and muscle tone.

The Merit of Vitamin E

An important corrective factor in all types of rheumatic ailment is vitamin E.

Considerable investigation into vitamin E has been carried out in the Arthritis Clinic, Rochester General Hospital, Rochester, USA by Dr C. L. Steinberg. Reporting in the *Annals of the New York Academy of Science*, he states that he gave vitamin E to 300 patients and relief from pain was obtained in the vast majority of cases. He recommended patients to keep on with a 'maintenance' dose after the symptoms have gone. He also treated rheumatic fever successfully with vitamin E.

Other doctors mentioned in the same journal have reported having used vitamin E for several different forms of rheumatism with great benefit to the patients, i.e. relief from pain, disappearance of physical symptoms and increased mobility of joints.

Considerable success in the treatment of rheumatic heart disease by the use of vitamin E is reported by Doctors W. E. and E. V. Shute in their book *Alpha Tocopherol (vitamin E) in Cardiovascular Disease.*

Vitamin E improves the whole circulatory mechanism. Blood is more freely carried to the muscles and joints affected by rheumatism or arthritis. In this way the acidity in the affected parts is more readily carried away and eliminated from the system in the normal way. Conversely, the curative elements are better circulated in the affected parts. Any factor that improves the blood supply inevitably improves the health in general and ailments in particular.

Dr E. Tuttle, a New York physician, told a British Commonwealth Medical Congress that osteoarthritis is not only simple wear and tear on the joints, as had been long thought. It starts with a deficiency of oxygen in the cell and then goes on to destroy the cell.

Vitamin E is most beneficial in ensuring the cell receives adequate oxygen. It does this by decreasing the oxygen requirement by almost 50 per cent, which is equivalent to increasing the normal flow of blood by the same amount. Vitamin E not only conserves oxygen, but strengthens muscular tissue as well. It also increases very considerably the curative effect of vitamin A. To obtain the maximum benefit, one vitamin E 100 i.u. capsule should be taken three times daily with meals.

Vitamin B_{12}

Vitamin B_{12} (one of the B complex vitamins) has produced good results in the treatment of osteoarthritis and spondylitis. However, this vitamin is found virtually only in foods of animal origin so vegetarians and vegans must look to a supplementary source to ensure an adequate intake. Usually 10 mcg per day taken with food is sufficient, but treatment of an arthritic condition may require more. High doses (1000 mcg) of vitamin B_{12} can only be introduced by intramuscular injection since the capacity of the body to absorb the vitamin from the intestine is very limited.

Lecithin and Rheumatic Diseases

Lecithin helps to diffuse blood calcium through the cell membrane, increases blood iodine and assists in the assimilation of organic phosphorus. It is also needed for the formation of healthy collagen (which is part of the connective tissues, cartilage and bone) according to the Lee Foundation for Nutritional Research, Milwaukee, USA.

It is significant that rheumatic and arthritic ailments are most prevalent in highly civilized countries where food processing and the hydrogenation of dietary fats are the norm. Such processing robs food of its lecithin content.

A typical daily intake of lecithin needed to prevent or to treat arthritis is a teaspoonful of the granules with each meal. Two high-potency lecithin capsules with each meal may suffice for some people, particularly if it is taken with vitamin E.

Calcium and Arthritis

Calcium is needed by every cell in the body: 98 per cent of the body's calcium is contained in the bones and teeth, and the nerves, muscles, and various organs all depend for their health on healthy bones. Calcium is essential to muscular health and a lack of calcium can give rise to cramps and convulsions. The heart is a muscle and needs calcium to regulate its rhythmic beat.

Is there any danger of getting too much calcium? With all the talk nowadays about calcification some people think that ingesting too much calcium may cause arthritis. The fact is that the body is excreting calcium continuously and the danger of obtaining too much calcium is an extremely remote possibility. In fact, the Australian diet is very likely to be deficient in calcium, according to Professor Sir Stanton Hicks, an eminent nutritional scientist.

Dr L. W. Cromwell of San Diego, California, reported to the Gerontological Society of San Francisco that he had found calcium deficiency to be a cause of arthritic crippling. This deficiency, he said, leads first to osteoporosis (loss of bone substance). Then, owing to depletion of bone calcium, the body compensates by depositing extra calcium at the points of greatest stress — the joints — which gives rise to increased structural rigidity at the joints.

A regular consumption of calcium tablets can help to correct both the osteoporotic condition mentioned above and the deposit of extra calcium around the bone joints which causes the stiffness and swelling of arthritis.

An Ideal Day's Diet

An ideal diet for someone who suffers from rheumatism would be on the following lines:

Before breakfast: A glass of diluted orange or lemon juice (no sugar).

Breakfast: Three to four dessertspoonfuls of wheatgerm, with milk, raisins and honey, or with grated apple and milk. Finish with grapes, if available, or stewed apricots, or prunes.

Mid-morning: Fruit juice, or cup of weak tea with thin slice of bread and butter.

Lunch: 2oz (50g) of unprocessed cheese and two or three apples, or celery. Celery is a good source of potassium and sodium and can help in rheumatic ailments. No bread-stuffs. Cheese is the one protein you require. It is a first-class source of amino acids for tissue replacement, and is rich in organic calcium, essential for healthy bones, cartilage and nerves.

Afternoon: Cup of weak tea, with slice of wholemeal bread, butter and honey.

Evening meal: Large greenleaf salad, milk and fruit. This should be preceded by a plate of hot, freshly-prepared vegetable soup in cold weather.

Before retiring: Take a dessertspoonful of molasses which can be thinned with a little hot water, if preferred. Molasses is rich in iron, which rheumatic sufferers lack.

This diet can be varied with discretion — some of the raw foods listed earlier can be included. A meal of meat, fish or eggs and vegetables is allowed two or three times per week.

Vitamin Supplementation
The following vitamin supplements should be taken with each meal:

Breakfast: Vitamin C 100 mg
Vitamin E 100 i.u.
Vitamin B complex (50 mg potency)

Lunch: Multimineral tablets (3 amino acid chelated)
Calcium pantothenate tablet (100 mg)
Vitamin C 100 mg
Vitamin E 100 i.u.

Dinner: Teaspoonful cod liver oil
Teaspoonful lecithin granules
Vitamin C 100 mg

This combination of supplements will help prevent arthritis if taken with a suitable diet. Higher potencies are required to treat a pre-existing condition and these are explained in the text.

5

Natural Treatments for Arthritis

In the previous chapter we discussed how diets and the sensible use of supplements can help prevent the development of rheumatic conditions. We shall now consider the latest natural treatments of these diseases for those individuals who already have them. All of these treatments have been subjected to some clinical trials and whilst the numbers of people involved do not compare with those using the orthodox treatments discussed in Chapter 3, many have found relief. The important advantage of these natural, alternative therapies is that side effects are virtually absent.

Pantothenic Acid (Calcium Pantothenate)

Early indications of a connection between pantothenic acid and arthritis came from studies on rats. When rats were deprived of the vitamin the young animals developed joint inflammation and impairment of hardening of the bones. These observations supported other studies that indicated that lack of pantothenic acid caused dogs and pigs to develop arthritic symptoms similar to those seen in human beings.

According to an article in *The Lancet* in 1963, blood pantothenic acid levels were measured in various groups of people, with and without arthritis. What emerged was that vegetarians have much higher blood levels of the vitamin than meat-eaters. This bears out the hypothesis that a vegetarian diet is less likely to cause arthritis.

All arthritic patients, whether vegetarian or not, had one common factor — greatly reduced levels of blood pantothenic acid. In fact, the lower the level of the vitamin in the blood, the more severe were the symptoms of the disease.

The two authors, Drs E. C. Barton-Wright and W. A. Elliott, then proceeded to test their hypothesis that arthritis is a pantothenic acid-deficient disease by treating their arthritic patients with daily injections of 50 mg calcium pantothenate. Royal jelly, a very rich source of the vitamin, was also given orally. Within seven days, the blood levels of pantothenic acid increased and these were parallelled by alleviation of the arthritic symptoms. This level of improvement did not change for a further three weeks on pantothenic acid treatment. However, once the treatment was stopped, the symptoms returned at their original intensity.

Following this initial encouraging report, Dr Arnaud reported in the same journal that he had noted relief of symptoms in patients suffering from osteoarthritis after small doses of calcium pantothenate.

Some years later, a much larger trial of the use of the vitamin in arthritis was undertaken by the General Practioner Research Group and reported in the journal *The Practioner* in 1980. A total of 94 patients were treated and neither they nor the doctors involved knew whether the treatment was calcium pantothenate or a harmless placebo. Response to the treatment was assessed both by doctor and patient using a number of criteria.

The dosage regime used was 500 mg (one tablet) daily for two days; 1000 mg (two tablets) for three days; 1500 mg (three tablets) for four days and finally 2000 mg (four tablets) per day thereafter for a period of two months. Calcium pantothenate-treated patients were found to have a reduced amount of morning stiffness, a lower degree of disability and a reduction in pain.

Only patients suffering from rheumatoid arthritis reported any significant benefit — there was little if any in other types of arthritis. No one is sure why pantothenic acid causes this improvement but one reason could be its involvement in the synthesis of the anti-stress hormones of the adrenal cortex. Lack of this vitamin could mean lowered production of these hormones with subsequent development of inflammatory and degenerative diseases like the arthritic conditions.

The ultimate treatment for these diseases, as we have seen, involves highly potent, synthetic hormones known as corticosteroids. Pantothenic acid may enable the glands of the body to produce their own, naturally-occuring corticosteroids. High potencies of the vitamin could be needed because the adrenals have become sluggish and not responsive to the ordinary quantities found in the diet. The end-result of either treatment is probably the same but of course the vitamin therapy is so much safer.

Vitamin A and Cod Liver Oil

Vitamin A acts upon the mucous membrane with which the inner surface of the body is lined. An example is the soft, pink tissue inside the mouth. Similar tissue covers the bronchial tubes, lungs, gall bladder, urinary bladder, sinuses, inside of ears and digestive tract, as well as the tubules in the kidneys.

When the diet is lacking in vitamin A, the body becomes especially susceptible to infectious diseases. Experiments carried out on laboratory animals reveal that those deprived of vitamin A in their diet develop diseases of the lungs, kidneys, bladder, nose and throat, sinuses, mastoids, ears, etc., while animals fed adequate amounts of vitamin A remain relatively free from such infections.

There is strong reason to believe that infections caused by lack of vitamin A provide suitable weakened conditions in the body for rheumatism or arthritis to manifest itself.

Cod liver oil has been promoted by Dr Dale Alexander as a treatment for arthritic conditions for many years. Undoubtedly some of the beneficial effects of this oil can be related to its vitamin A content, but recent research has suggested that some of the polyunsaturated fatty acids present in cod liver oil also contribute to its effectiveness.

The oil is particularly rich in two fatty acids called EPA (eicosapentaenoic acid) and DHA (docosahexaenoic acid). These acids are precursors of essential hormones in the body called prostaglandins and these have the ability to reduce the inflammation, swelling and degeneration associated with the various types of arthritis and rheumatism.

It is quite possible that in an arthritic joint, the body has lost the ability to produce these protective prostaglandins. Supplying their precursors in the form of cod liver oil appears to stimulate their production so they can then exert their beneficial effects where needed.

Sometimes a large quantity of cod liver oil is required, and since this also supplies high potencies of vitamins A and D there is the possibility of an overdose of these vitamins on prolonged treatment. This problem has now been overcome by the availability of cod liver oil that contains the necessary fatty acids EPA and DHA without the accompanying vitamins. Alternatively, concentrated fish-body oils that contain higher potencies of EPA and DHA can be taken in capsule form. The dosage is up to five capsules daily until relief is obtained; then they can be reduced to a daily number that maintains relief. A teaspoonful of cod liver oil with each meal is the alternative dose.

New Zealand Green-Lipped Mussel Extract

In his book *Natural Relief from Arthritis* (Thorsons, 1979) John Croft describes a safe and effective treatment for arthritic conditions that uses a simple extract of the particular green-lipped mussel that is confined to the waters around New Zealand. Controlled clinical trials using the extract carried out in hospitals have indicated a success rate in relieving the symptoms of arthritis comparable to that of potent, synthetic drugs: 70 per cent of rheumatoid arthritis patients and 40 per cent of osteoarthritis patients gained varying degrees of relief.

The usual regime is 1 gram of the green-lipped mussel extract daily, taken in three doses of 330 mg, each with a meal. Once relief is obtained, and it may take some weeks before it happens, the dosage may be reduced to that which maintains relief. In some arthritics, the condition may appear to worsen after ten days or so, but this simply means the treatment is working and it should be persevered with. Those with known allergies to shellfish should proceed with caution although as the treatment is an extract, even these people may be able to tolerate it.

New Zealand Green-Lipped Mussel Extract contains an anti-inflammatory agent but it may also have some effect upon the disease process. The identification of the active principle will soon be known and this could open up a new chapter in the treatment of arthritic conditions.

Devil's Claw
Devil's Claw is the popular name for *Harpagophytum Procumbens,* a plant found in the Kalahari Desert and in Namibia. The name derives from its appearance which is like a rosette that grows on the ground with eight finger-like outgrowths which are turned up and armed with thorns. Once dry the plants pose problems for animals who can be injured when they tread on them.

The roots are extracted with water and the aqueous extract is dried before being incorporated into tablets. Each tablet contains 410 mg of dried extract equivalent to 820 mg of the original root. In treating arthritis the usual dose is three tablets daily, one with each meal.

Typical of the many trials carried out on Devil's Claw is that of Professor Zorn of the University of Jena, USA. He found that after five weeks treatment the swelling was reduced and stiff joints became mobile again. In addition, relief of symptoms continued after a course of treatment had been completed. For this reason, a break of two weeks or so after a twenty-week treatment is usually recommended. A darkly-coloured urine is often noted during treatment with Devil's Claw. This is absolutely harmless and indicates that the body is purifying itself.

As an alternative to tablets, a tea infusion can be made from the herb in teabags. It is best to prepare it the evening before — one teabag with boiling water — to enable the infusion to draw out overnight and then to drink it the next day. One third of the liquid should be taken ten minutes before each meal. If the bitter taste is unacceptable, a tablet can be taken instead, 10 minutes before each meal.

Yucca Plant

A clinical trial reported in the *Journal of Applied Nutrition* (1975) from the National Arthritis Medical Clinic indicated that an extract of the desert yucca plant was beneficial in treating rheumatoid and osteoarthritis. The study was a double-blind one, meaning that neither patient nor doctor knew whether the treatment was yucca extract or a harmless placebo. Assessment was measured by subjective responses by the patients and by objective observations by the doctors: 165 patients were studied.

Patients took from two to eight tablets daily, with

an average of four. The period over which they were taken varied from one week to fifteen months. Tablets could be taken before, during or after meals with no problems either way on the gastrointestinal tract.

On assessing the beneficial effect, 49 per cent of patients reported favourably, 28 per cent felt there was no effect and 23 per cent were undecided. As to the major complaints of arthritis, 61 per cent felt less swelling, less pain and less stiffness; 39 per cent reported no change. Beneficial response was felt by some in an average of 3.5 days; some in an average of 2.3 weeks and the last group in an average of 3.2 months.

There were no reports of untoward effects. There were no allergic reactions reported nor observed and blood tests on the patients indicated no changes in normal values of the constituents. Those with high blood-cholesterol levels at the start of the trial showed reduced levels at the end of a few weeks treatment.

The main reason for lack of side effects is that the yucca saponin (the active constituent) is not absorbed from the intestine and indeed appears to exert its action there. It is likely that the saponin acts upon the friendly bacteria that live in the large intestine. Other studies suggest that the yucca extract contains another constituent with a mild anti-inflammatory action also.

Homoeopathic Remedies

Homoeopathy is a system of medicine developed by a German physician, Dr S. C. Hahnemann in the late eighteenth century. The principle of the system is 'like cures like' which means that a toxic substance that can give rise to a particular complaint, if given at doses that the individual can tolerate, will relieve the symptoms of that complaint.

Over the years Dr Hahnemann and others set themselves the task first of determining which natural substances that were also toxic gave rise to the symptoms of a particular disease. Once the minimum dose necessary to produce those symptoms was determined by experimentation on themselves, Dr Hahnemann and his colleagues then gave the same substances at the same low dosage to their patients. The result was that when the symptoms of the disease paralleled those of the treatment, relief was often obtained and the patients were effectively cured.

The system of homoeopathy is based upon three principles that are the basis of all treatments:

1 If a natural substance or medicine that produces symptoms of a disease in a normal healthy person is given to a sick person suffering from that disease, the symptoms of the illness are often relieved.

2 Once the natural substance or medicine is identified, it is diluted many times in order to enhance the properties of the medicine. There is the added advantage that such massive dilution also eliminates possible side effects.

3 The philosophy of homoeopathy is to treat the whole person, unlike conventional drugs which function in a specific manner on a particular part of the body and seek only to remove symptoms. Homoeopathy treats the basis of disease.

A fundamental belief of Dr Hahnemann was that the body has an in-built ability to heal itself — a function he recognized even before the discovery of antibodies that fight off infection. He suggested that symptoms of a disease were simply the reactions of the body to overcome that disease. Homoeopathic treatment merely encouraged the body to manifest its own healing processes. For these reasons homoeopathic remedies were safe, gentle medicines that assisted the body to ward off disease or treat a pre-existing one.

The twin secrets of homoeopathy are therefore identification of the specific active principle to treat the disease and determination of the most dilute solution of that principle that can be beneficial. Although it appears to go against all logic, the more a remedy is diluted the more effective it becomes according to homoeopathic principles.

The most popular dilution in homoeopathy is known as 6X. All this means is that an extract of the remedy, usually a herb or plant, is diluted in the ratio one part extract to 99 parts of an alcohol/water mixture. This is called 1X. One part of this diluted extract is mixed with a further 99 parts of the alcohol/water solvent to give the dilution 2X. One part of this 2X dilution is further diluted with 99 parts of solvent to give a 3X dilution and the process is carried on until the 6X dilution is obtained. At this infinitesimal concentration the active principle is given to the patient in liquid form. A similar process can be carried out in the dried form and the final dilution presented as a tablet. The dilutent here is usually a sugar. The tablets are usually placed upon the tongue and allowed to dissolve to ensure maximum absorption into the blood stream.

The specific homoeopathic remedy for rheumatism and allied conditions like arthritis, lumbago and sciatica is an alcoholic extract (or tincture) of the fresh leaves of the Poison Ivy plant also known as *Rhus toxicodendron*. The 6X preparation is taken orally in tablet form and may also be incorporated into an ointment for direct application to the affected area. There are many cases on record of this treatment providing relief from the symptoms of rheumatic conditions. Even less painful conditions like sprains and athletic injuries often respond to the homoeopathic ointment alone. Since they are so safe, homoeopathic tablets of Rhus can be taken as often as desired but the best treatment is that suggested on the pack since this regimen has been proved by experience. The ointment can be applied by gentle massage as often as is necessary but particularly before going to bed, as rheumatic pains often become worse at night.

Tissue Salts
Dr W. H. Schuessler was the first to put forward the theory that any tissue salt deficiency, or imbalance, results in disease. He suggested that by supplying the tissue salt which is lacking, the body cells can again function normally and health is restored.

According to the theory of Dr Schuessler there are twelve tissue salts (or mineral salts) present in the blood and cells of the body and they are the key factors in the normal, healthy metabolism of these cells. All twelve tissue salts must be present in the correct proportions in order to create normal body cells and to maintain them in a healthy state.

On the basis of his observations and experimentation, Dr Schuessler proposed five principles on which his biochemic remedies hinge:

1 Disease does not occur if cell metabolism is normal.
2 Cell metabolism is normal only if cell nutrition is adequate.
3 All nutritional substances are either of an organic or an inorganic nature if they are to be utilized by the body.
4 The ability of body cells to assimilate and metabolize nutritional substances is impaired if there is any deficiency of a tissue salt.
5 Adequate cell nutrition can be restored and cell metabolism brought back to normal by simply supplying the required tissue salts to the depleted cells.

An important aspect of restoring tissue salts to body cells is that they must be supplied in a very finely divided form. This is to ensure efficient and total absorption followed by rapid and complete assimilation. The tissue salts are diluted in accordance with homoeopathic principles (see previous section) before being presented as solutions or as tablets but here the similarity with homoeopathy ends. Tissue salts are only twelve in number and all are minerals but homoeopathy utilizes dozens of herbal and other remedies and functions on different principles.

The biochemical functions of the tissue salts are as follows:

Calc. Fluor (calcium fluoride) — maintains tissue elasticity. Deficiency causes loss of elasticity or an over-relaxed tissue, particularly in muscles and joints.

Calc. Phos. (calcium phosphate) — essential component of bones, teeth and gastric juices and so benefits the digestive systems and can be used to treat teething problems and chilblains.

Calc. Sulph. (calcium sulphate) — blood constituent that speeds up the healing process and hence acts to clear up minor skin complaints.

Ferr. Phos. (ferrous phosphate) — functions in the oxygenation of the blood stream. Relieves coughs and feverish colds.

Kali. Mur. (potassium chloride) — normally used alternately with Ferr. Phos. in relieving minor respiratory disorders, particularly those of children.

Kali. Phos. (potassium phosphate) — functions as a nerve soother. Used to treat overactive nerves, nervous headache and nervous indigestion.

Kali. Sulph. (potassium sulphate) — necessary to maintain a healthy skin so it is used to treat skin conditions. Has been used to relieve catarrh.

Mag. Phos. (magnesium phosphate) — used to treat minor pains and muscular cramps. Relieves flatulence.

Nat. Mur. (sodium chloride) — controls water levels of the body and helps to prevent excessive watery secretions like those suffered in respiratory complaints. Has been used to treat loss of smell or taste.

Nat. Phos. (sodium phosphate) — functions as acid neutralizer — particularly needed for relief of excess gastric acid and heartburn. Has been used to relieve rheumatic pain when this is due to too much acidity.

Nat. Sulph. (sodium sulphate) — like Nat. Mur. controls water balance of the body. Used to treat digestive upsets and influenza.

Silica — functions as cleanser and conditioner. Hence used to clear up minor skin blemishes. Alternates with Kali. Sulph. in treating brittle nails.

Arthritis and related conditions are usually treated according to the following tissue salts regimens.

Arthritis
Ferr. Phos. Relieves acute attacks of fever and swollen, inflammatory joints.

Nat. Phos. Neutralizes excess acid when this is the cause of the condition. May be used alternately with Nat. Sulph.

Nat. Mur. Used specifically to relieve creaking joints.

Mag. Phos. When used alternately with Calc. Phos. can relieve the pain of osteoarthritis.

All four tissue salts are available in combination tablets.

Fibrositis
Ferr. Phos. The main remedy for acute pains of inflammation brought on suddenly by chills, exercise,

strains and exposure to the cold.

Kali. Sulph. Tends to be used to relieve fleeting or shifting pains.

Mag. Phos. Has been used to relieve the sharp, spasmodic pains associated with the condition.

All three are available as a combination tablet.

Gout
Ferr. Phos. Used to relieve fever and the inflammatory stage of the condition.

Nat. Sulph. Neutralizes the effects of the rich foods that can bring on gout. Also relieves any bilious symptoms present due to the same cause. In an acute attack can be used alternately with Ferr. Phos.

Nat. Phos. Neutralizes the excess uric acid which is one of the causes of the condition.

Lumbago
Ferr. Phos. Relieves the pain, fever, and inflammation associated with the early stages.

Nat. Phos. Neutralizes the acidity causing the condition.

Calc. Phos. Relieves the backache and stiffness, particularly that suffered on waking.

Calc. Fluor. Should be used to relieve any back pain that follows a strain.

Nat. Mur. Used to relieve the pain induced by prolonged stooping, that caused by lying on a hard surface, and the sensation of coldness in the spine.

Available as a specific combination tablet.

Rheumatism
Ferr. Phos. Relieves the pain, fever, heat, redness and fast pulse associated with the first stages of a rheumatic attack.

Kali. Mur. Relieves the second stage of rheumatism where swelling of the affected part has developed. Can be alternated with Ferr. Phos.

Nat. Phos. An important remedy that neutralizes the excess acidity that gives rise to acid perspiration, acid taste in the mouth and a yellow coating on the tongue that are associated with the condition.

Nat. Sulph. Aids in the removal of toxic substances from the body.

Silica Acts by removing the uric acid that has crystallized in the joints and muscles.

Calc. Phos. Should be used for rheumatism that becomes worse at night or is brought on by cold weather, wet weather or other environmental change.

Calc. Fluor. Reduces the swelling of the joints that is a feature of some stages of rheumatism.

Mag. Phos. Relieves the sharp, spasmodic pains, often excruciating, that are a feature of rheumatism.

All these tissue salts are available as a specific combination.

Sciatica
Ferr. Phos. Used mainly to relieve early pain and inflammation.

Mag. Phos. Treats the pain when it is spasmodic.

Kali. Phos. Alternates with Mag. Phos. to relieve nervous exhaustion that is associated with the restlessness that is a feature of the condition.

Nat. Sulph. Used to relieve the pain induced by any sort of movement.

Bursitis (also known as synovitis)
Ferr. Phos. Used mainly to relieve early pain, inflammation and stiffness.

Nat. Sulph. Removes the excess water causing swelling of the joint.

Silica Used mainly in relief of the chronic condition where there is swelling and difficulty in moving.

Calc. Fluor. Tends to be taken when the condition is long standing and is resistant to other treatments.

Like homoeopathic remedies, Biochemic Tissue Salts are completely non-toxic. They are most beneficial however when used exactly as suggested on the pack. Presentation of tissue salts is usually as small tablets which dissolve readily on the tongue and are quickly absorbed and assimilated.

Herbal Remedies
The various herbs used to treat arthritic and rheumatic conditions function in many ways. Some

act as diuretics to promote the flow of urine and hence rid the body of poisons; some are purgatives to clear the bowel of toxic substances believed to be responsible for rheumatism; others contain anti-inflammatory agents to reduce the pain and swelling of inflamed joints; some increase the flow of blood to and from the affected tissues to help clear away accumulated toxins.

Although individual herbs possess one or more of these properties, the most effective preparations for relieving arthritis and rheumatism are those containing carefully selected combinations of herbs that will contribute to all aspects of the healing process. Most herbal preparations are taken orally but there are herbs that act topically on the affected areas in the form of ointments and creams. As well as tablets and capsules, there are also available herbal teas that can help relieve the symptoms of rheumatic conditions.

Let us now look at some of the more specific herbal remedies:

Aconitum — known also as Monkshood, Wolfsbane
Contains numerous alkaloids that have a pain-killing and muscle-relaxing action. Can only be used in ointment or cream for direct application to the painful area. On no account to be taken orally. Usual strength for application is a 1.3 per cent lotion or 1 part tincture to 9 parts Witch Hazel.
Specific for rheumatic pain, sciatica.

Apium — celery fruit or seed
Acts as an anti-rheumatic agent and sedative for relaxing the affected areas. Useful when rheumatic

condition is associated with mild depression. Most effective when combined with Menyanthes and Guaiacum; the therapeutic action is potentiated by Taraxacum (Dandelion).
Usual dose of Apium is 0.5-2.0 g, three times daily. Specific for arthritis, gout, rheumatism.

Bryonia — White Bryony, Wild Vine
Can be used in direct application as ointment and in small doses as oral preparation. Oral doses should not be more than 0.5 g three times daily. Specific for rheumatic pain and lumbago. Large internal doses may precipitate menstruation or cause haemorrhoids. Avoid during pregnancy.

Capsicum — Cayenne, African Chillies
Best used externally as a lotion or ointment in treating lumbago and rheumatic pains.

Castanea — Sweet Chestnut
Has been used in combination with Apium, Cimifuga, Menyanthes and Filipendula in muscular rheumatism and fibrositis. Usual dose is 2-4 g dried leaf, three times daily.

Cimifuga — Black Cohosh, Black Snakeroot, Actaeae Racemosae Radix
Contains salicylic acid which is a natural anti-inflammatory agent and pain-killer. Usual dose is 0.3 to 2 g of the dried root, three times daily.
Specific for muscular rheumatism and rheumatoid arthritis. Most efficient when taken with Menyanthes or Apium.

Devil's Claw — see p. 84-5.

Dioscorea — Wild Yam Root, Colic Root, Rheumatism Root

Contains steroid glycosides which probably contribute to its anti-rheumatic action. Combines well with Cimifuga in rheumatoid arthritis.

Specific for the acute phase of rheumatoid arthritis. Indicated also for the chronic condition and for muscular rheumatism.

Usual dose is 2-4g of the dried root three times daily.

Filipendula — Meadow Sweet, *Spiraea ulmaria*

The herb is a rich source of salicylic compounds and bioflavonoids which are analgesic and anti-inflammatory.

Has been used to treat rheumatic muscle and joint pains but is more effective with other herbs such as Gaultheria and Guaiacum.

Usual dose is 4-6g of the dried herb, three times daily.

Gaultheria — Wintergreen, Teaberry, Checkerberry

Active constituent is oil of Wintergreen or Methyl Salicylate which has analgesic properties and stimulates blood flow to affected area. Usual oral dose is 0.5-1.0 g dried leaves, three times daily. The oil is available in ointments for topical application. Specific for rheumatoid arthritis but also used to relieve sciatica. Best combined with Filipendula and Menyanthes in treating rheumatic conditions.

Guaiacum — *Lignum vitae*, Guaiac

Contains substances with diuretic, laxative and anti-rheumatic properties. Induces sweating. Usual oral dose is 1-2 g of the dried wood, three times daily. Specific for chronic rheumatism and rheumatoid arthritis but taken regularly can prevent recurrence of gout. Best combined with Menyanthes, Filipendula and Apium.

Hypericum — Common St John's Wort
Contains astringents, bioflavonoids and a volatile oil which are analgesic and sedative. Usual dose is 2-4 g dried herb, three times daily.
Specific for fibrositis and sciatica both in the oral form and as a topical ointment.

Jacobaea — Common Ragwort, St James's Wort
Contains anti-inflammatory glycosides and bioflavonoids. Used only as a topical treatment. The lotion is usually a 1 in 5 extract in 10 per cent alcohol. Specific for rheumatoid arthritis, rheumatism and sciatica but is better combined with Gaultheria and Lobelia.

Lappa — Burdock Herb (root)
Contains bitters and bioflavonoids that act as diuretics. Usual dose is 2-6 g dried root or herb, three times daily.
Indicated in rheumatism and gout.

Lobelia — Indian Tobacco
When incorporated into an ointment it is used to remove the pain of rheumatic nodules.

Menyanthes — Bogbean, Buckbean, Marsh Trefoil
Contains active glycosides and bitters that act as diuretics. Combines well with Apium or Cimifuga in relieving muscular rheumatism. Usual dose is 1-2 g dried leaves, three times daily.
Indicated for rheumatism and rheumatoid arthritis.

Populus — Quaking Aspen, White Poplar
Contains salicin, a natural analgesic and anti-inflammatory similar in action to aspirin. Best used with Cimifuga and Menyanthes to treat rheumatoid arthritis. Usual dose is 1-4 g dried herb, three times daily.
Specific for rheumatoid arthritis but used extensively for muscular rheumatism.

Salix — Willow, Willow Bark
Rich source of salicin, a natural analgesic and anti-inflammatory agent. Also reduces high body temperature. Usual dose is 1-3 g dried bark, three times daily.
Specific for rheumatoid arthritis and any inflammatory rheumatic condition. Often used with Cimifuga, Apium and Guaiacum in rheumatoid arthritis. Indications include muscular rheumatism, gouty arthritis and ankylosing spondylitis.

Sassafras — Cinnamon Wood, Ague Tree, Saloop, Sassafras Root Bark, Saxifrax
Contains diuretic and anti-inflammatory agents. The oil is suitable only for topical use. Usual dose is 2-4 g dried bark, three times daily.
Specific for rheumatic pains and gout.

Zanthoxylum Bark — Prickly Ash Bark, Toothache Bark, Xanthoxylum
Increases blood flow in rheumatic conditions. Used usually with Guaiacum, Menyanthes and Capsicum in rheumatism. Usual dose is 1-3 g dried bark, three times daily.

6

The Sweat Therapy

The human body makes use of fevers as a natural
method of loosening and expelling poisonous and
waste substances. A fever is thus a powerful curative
agency, for by its heat it also burns up bacteria and
their poisons.

A local inflammation is actually a local fever in
which the affected tissue is trying to rid itself of toxic
matter. By inducing sweating artificially, a rise in
temperature can be produced that has similar curative
properties to fever. Copious perspiration rids the
body not only of the usual waste products of
perspiration — i.e. water, acids, salts, etc. — but also
of poisonous matter which is causing sickness or
retarding recovery. This is why various ways of
inducing perspiration have long been used
successfully in rheumatic ailments. These sweating
methods have the additional advantage of relieving
pain.

Let us now review some of the simplest methods of
inducing perspiration.

Walking
The patient dresses in warm woollen underclothes

and over it wears warm clothing and an overcoat. He or she now takes a long vigorous walk in the sun. After half an hour or so he or she will begin to perspire freely, and this can be kept up as long as required. At first the patient will feel oppressively hot, but once sweating starts and the poisonous matter begins to be expelled, there is a feeling of strength.

The patient should then return home, undress quickly, take a cool shower, and go to bed. This treatment should be kept up for several days in succession. In dull weather, a hot lemon drink should be taken before commencing the walk.

This therapy is obviously unsuitable for those with high blood-pressure or heart ailments.

Bed Sweating

If the patient for any reason is unfit to induce perspiration by walking, he or she should be wrapped in a dry sheet and one or two blankets (the arms should be able to move, although they are covered). Hot water bottles should be placed at the feet and on each side of the body and hot lemon drinks given. The patient should begin to perspire profusely after half an hour or so. The period of sweating should be followed by a cool shower and then back to bed. Alternatively, the patient can be given a rub down with a towel dipped in tepid water.

Steam Baths

A simple steam bath can be taken at home using a stool or kitchen chair, beneath which one or more containers of boiling water are placed. The patient sits down and a sheet and several blankets are placed around him or her (leaving the head free) so that the steam cannot escape. As a container of water cools another one with boiling water should be substituted. The first bath should not exceed twenty minutes and as many as two or three steam baths a week may be taken.

Partial steam baths

These may be taken for lumbago, sciatica and rheumatism around the hips. Proceed as for an ordinary steam bath, but drape the sheet and blankets no higher than the hips, and cover the upper part of the body, where no steam can reach, to keep it warm.

A partial steam bath for the head and chest is beneficial in rheumatism of the shoulder joints, between the ribs, and the chest muscles. The patient sits facing another chair back and leans the upper part of his or her body over a vessel of hot water. He or she is covered with a blanket so that no steam can escape. A cool shower should be taken after the bath, which should not last longer than ten to fifteen minutes.

A partial steam bath can be taken for legs and feet by those with rheumatism in the lower limbs, gout, or inflammation of the knee. The container of boiling water is placed near a low stool upon which the legs are rested, and covered with a blanket to retain the steam. After the bath, the legs and feet should be washed and then rested with the legs raised.

Benefits of steam baths

When the body is exposed to steam, the temperature of the blood rises and the heat is transmitted to inner organs. The circulation of the blood and the heart's rhythmic action are thereby stimulated and the blood pressure rises.

Sweating should occur after a few minutes' exposure to steam, but in some instances thirty or more minutes may be needed to induce copious perspiration. An intense perspiration should be sought as this provides maximum benefits, not only for the skin, which as an organ of elimination contains many millions of functioning pores, but also for the kidneys, liver and lungs. Perspiration can be increased during the bath by hot lemon drinks. After the steam bath, a tepid shower should be taken and the patient should go to bed.

Because of their effect upon the blood pressure, steam baths should not be taken by those with severe heart ailments or high blood pressure, nor should they be continued for extended periods by anyone, as they tire the heart.

Hot and Cold Baths

Hot water causes tense and stiffened muscles, joints, and ligaments to relax. It also promotes the circulation of blood through congested areas where pain is located. Every hot bath should be followed by a cold shower. The cold water prevents the hot bath from having an enervating effect upon the skin. Cold water, applied in moderation to the skin, has a tonic effect, causing blood to return to the surface and speeding up the circulation. A quick rub down after the cold shower restores vitality both to the skin and the nerve endings just beneath it.

Water Compresses

The damp pack or water compress is applied by wringing out a bed sheet in lukewarm or cool water and spreading it over two blankets. The patient is laid on the damp sheet, which is folded around him or her. The two blankets should then be folded separately and neatly around the patient and a quilt placed on top. The head should be placed in a comfortable posture.

A sheet of plastic material, or even several sheets of newspaper, placed below the dampened bedsheet will prevent the mattress from becoming wet. The body, after the intial sensation of coldness, soon begins to glow. As the compress warms up, the patient will experience a soothing, pleasurable feeling; pain is relieved and a profuse perspiration commences. If the patient falls off to sleep, do not disturb him or her but after he or she awakes a tepid or cool shower should be taken to remove impurities adhering to the skin, and the patient should then return to bed.

The Leg Pack

This pack is useful for rheumatism or arthritis in the leg, for gout, and for varicose veins. The easiest way to apply it is to wring out thin stockings in cold water, put them on each leg and then over the top draw on thick dry woollen stockings. Both legs should be done together, not just the affected leg. This pack is very effective in absorbing poisonous substances from the legs.

Damp packs of a similar nature can be used for the ankles, knees, hands, wrists and arms, whenever there is pain or inflammation.

Hot Epsom Salts Baths

To speed up the elimination of uric acid from the system, it is important to induce its excretion through the pores. A hot Epsom salts bath will do this and can be taken twice weekly as follows: dissolve 1 lb of commercial Epsom salts in boiling water, and add to a hot bath, one-third full. Remain immersed in the bath for ten minutes. This bath should be taken before going to bed, but take care not to get chilled afterwards. Do not use soap with the Epsom salts bath as it interferes with its beneficial effects.

Epsom salts (magnesium sulphate) has a strong affinity for carbon, which explains its value for medicinal purposes. For carbon, in one form or another, is the main constituent of the building materials which go to form our vegetation and so, in turn, to provide our foodstuffs, and it is in the crude form of carbon that the waste products of the human body are thrown off. The magnesium draws out the carbon and renders the now inert residue soluble, thereby facilitating its excretion.

The chief value of Epsom salts lies in its external application because of its power of drawing uric acid waste from the body through the pores of the skin.

Those who are frail and weak should begin with a small quantity, such as ½lb of Epsom salts and then gradually increase the amount as the bath becomes better tolerated. These baths are not advised for anyone with a heart condition or high blood pressure. The bath water should not be hotter than bloodheat (98.6°F, 38.6°C).

7
Final Word

Short periods of pain and stiffness lasting just a few days or weeks are distressing at the time but are eventually forgotten. Even a displaced disc may cause severe backache for a time but it may disappear completely and never return. There are however some backaches and pains in neck, shoulders, arms and legs that may persist, making life a misery. This chronic condition is that which most people will endure if they develop arthritic disease.

The question of how much exercise should an arthritic take is constantly being asked since, as we have seen, some exercise is essential. If feet, ankles, knees or hips are painfully affected, it is best to restrict physical exertion that involves much walking or running. A degree of mobility has to be maintained and the joints must be exercised daily but prolonged bouts of exercise should be avoided. If exertion causes the pain or swelling in a joint to increase for two hours or more afterwards, it is a warning that you have exercised too much. Cutting down on the exercise will prevent this after effect and you are your

own best judge as to the amount you can really
tolerate.

The rheumatic sufferer, armed with the information
set out in this book, is able to work out his or her own
salvation from rheumatism in any of its forms. All
that you need in addition to this information is the
will to persevere and the commonsense to understand
that a deep-seated arthritic condition that has
probably taken fifty years to create, cannot be cured in
a month. Many months of faithful and intelligent
application of the corrective principles and nutrition
are necessary before deep-seated arthritic conditions
begin to disappear. We have known some of the most
distorted cases — cases given up by the hospitals as
incurable — to improve considerably. One further
thing is certain: rheumatism will seldom occur or
return while you adhere to the remedial principles
outlined in this book.

It may take three months for your system to adapt
itself to these principles, but it will take six to twelve
months before you see any substantial improvement
in your arthritic condition. (Simpler forms of
rheumatism usually improve in from two to six
months.) In two years, however, the most obstinate
cases of rheumatoid or osteoarthritis should show
definite signs of improvement; and long before this
the pain should have eased and your general health be
greatly improved. From that point onwards your
progress lies in your own hands. It is all a matter of
how consistently and intelligently you apply the
corrective measures day after day, month after month,
and year after year.

The prospect of a long struggle to regain health will

deter all but the most determined from making the effort;.but those who do will reap life's richest reward — improved health.

Index